Silence the Voices

Books from the Institute for the Study of Peak States

Peak States of Consciousness: Theory and Applications, Volume 1: Breakthrough Techniques for Exceptional Quality of Life, by Dr. Grant McFetridge with Jacquelyn Aldana and Dr. James Hardt (2004)

Peak States of Consciousness: Theory and Applications, Volume 2: Acquiring Extraordinary Spiritual and Shamanic States by Grant McFetridge Ph.D. with Wes Gietz (2008)

Peak States of Consciousness: Theory and Applications, Volume 3: Subcellular Psychobiology, Disease, and Immunity by Grant McFetridge Ph.D., et al. (forthcoming)

The Basic Whole-Hearted Healing™ Manual (3rd Edition) by Grant McFetridge Ph.D. and Mary Pellicer M.D. (2004)

The Whole-Hearted Healing™ Workbook by Paula Courteau (2013)

Subcellular Psychobiology Diagnosis Handbook: Subcellular Causes of Psychological Symptoms - Peak States® Therapy, Volume 1 by Grant McFetridge Ph.D. (2014)

Silence the Voices: Discovering the Biology of Mind Chatter - Peak States® Therapy, Volume 2 by Grant McFetridge Ph.D. (2017)

Addiction and Withdrawal - Peak States® Therapy, Volume 3 by Kirsten Lykkegaard Ph.D. and Grant McFetridge Ph.D. (forthcoming)

Suicide Prevention - Peak States® Therapy, Volume 4 by Thomas Gagey M.D. and Grant McFetridge Ph.D. (forthcoming)

Spiritual Emergencies - Peak States® Therapy, Volume 5 by Grant McFetridge Ph.D. and Nemi Nath (forthcoming)

Breakthrough Research: Techniques, Insights, and Mindset by Grant McFetridge Ph.D. et al. (forthcoming)

Silence the Voices

Discovering the Biology of Mind Chatter

Peak States® Therapy, Volume 2

By Grant McFetridge Ph.D.
Illustrations by Piotr Kawecki and Lorenza Meneghini

Foreword: Working in Research
By Thomas Gagey, M.D.

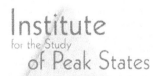

Institute
for the Study
of Peak States

"Methods for Fundamental Change in the Human Psyche"

First Edition
First Printing, 2017
ISBN 978-0-9734680-9-0

Cataloguing-in-Publication Data

McFetridge, Grant T., 1955-
Silence the voices: Discovering the biology of mind chatter / by Grant McFetridge; foreword by Thomas Gagey.
p. cm.
Includes bibliographical references and index.
ISBN 978-0-9734680-9-0 (soft cover)

1. Schizophrenia—Treatment.   2.Developmental biology.
3. Psychobiology—Subcellular. 4. Psychoneuroimmunology. 5. Mycosis.
I. McFetridge, Grant T. II. Title.
362.26 –dc21

The following are trademarks of the Institute for the Study of Peak States: Peak States®, Whole-Hearted Healing®, Silent Mind Technique™, Body Association Technique™, Tribal Block Technique™, Triune Brain Therapy™, and the Courteau Projection Technique™.

Institute for the Study of Peak States
3310 Cowie Rd, Hornby Island, BC
V0R 1Z0 Canada
http://www.PeakStates.com

*This book is dedicated to all the individuals who helped
make these discoveries possible, especially:*

Florence Mary-Martha McFetridge RN, and John S. McFetridge MD
*To my parents who were my biggest fans,
your loving encouragement has always been with me,*

and

Steve and Jessie Hsu
*My dear friends and colleagues,
whose enthusiasm and financial support made this book a reality.*

Legal Liability Agreement
IMPORTANT!
READ THE FOLLOWING BEFORE CONTINUING WITH THE TEXT

The material in this book is provided for educational purposes only, and is *not* intended to be used by the general public as a self-help aid. The processes in this book are for the benefit of professionals in the field of trauma healing, and are not meant to be used by lay people without *competent and qualified supervision*. As this is a relatively new and specialized field of study, even most licensed professionals do not have adequate background and training in both prenatal and perinatal psychology and power therapies.

It is possible, and in some cases probable that you will feel extreme distress, both short and long term, if you use the processes in this book. As with any intense psychological process, life-threatening problems might occur due to the possibility of stressing a weak heart, from activating suicidal feelings, and other causes. Although we've explicitly indicated in the text the potential problems that you might encounter using these processes, you may encounter something we haven't seen before. You may experience serious or life-threatening problems with any of the processes in this book. The possibility that you may die from using these processes *does* exist. If you are not willing to be TOTALLY responsible for how you use this material, and any consequences to doing so, then we require that you not use the processes in this book. This should be obvious, but we wanted to make it totally explicit.

Given what we've just said, the following common sense statements constitute a legal agreement between us. This applies to everyone, including licensed professionals and lay people. Please read the following statements carefully:

1. The author, any people associated with the Institute for the Study of Peak States, and other contributors to this text cannot and will not take responsibility for what you do with the material in this book and these techniques.
2. You are required to take complete responsibility for your own emotional and physical well-being if you use these processes or any variations of them.
3. You are required to instruct others on whom you use these processes, or variations of these processes, that they are completely responsible for their own emotional and physical well-being.
4. Use these techniques under the supervision of a qualified therapist or physician as appropriate.
5. You must agree to hold harmless the author and anyone associated with this text or with the Institute for the Study of Peak States from any claims made by anyone, yourself included, on whom you use these processes, or variations of them.
6. Many of the process names in this book are trademarked, and so the usual legal restrictions apply to their public use.

Out of consideration for the safety of others:
- You are required to instruct other people on whom you use these processes or variations of these processes of the dangers involved, and that they are completely responsible for their own emotional and physical wellbeing.
- If you write (or communicate in other ways) to others about the new and experimental material in this book, you agree to inform them that there are possible dangers involved with working with this material, and to give specifics where applicable.

Continuing with this text constitutes a legal agreement to these conditions. Thank you for your understanding.

Contents

Appendices

Foreword: Working in Research

by Thomas Gagey, M.D. (Psychiatry)

This book is mainly focused on the question of hearing voices, but it will also give you a fascinating insight about the research made by Dr. Grant McFetridge and his colleagues for more than 20 years.

In this book, you will discover lots of techniques, some of which are working specifically with voices and you will understand how they were invented.

In the last chapter, you will get more information about a new, simpler process that is currently being tested (by myself and others) to treat voices. I really hope that testing on a larger amount of people will confirm its efficiency and stability. In this case, I believe it can be a very helpful tool that could be added to those that are already working to decrease the suffering of people that hear voices

I wish you an exciting exploration in this field…

The discomfort of exploring something new

I was in the middle of my medical school when I first heard about Grant and the Institute for the Study of Peak States (ISPS). At that time, I was interested in psychology and hypnosis; I was reading a post on a hypnosis forum when I came across a guy describing the value of ISPS methods.

I remember well my gut feeling, a kind of "seems strange but I want to know more".

And so I bought Grant's first volume about peak states of consciousness and started to read it. On one hand, I was feeling excited as it described some very interesting states I had experienced while in self-hypnosis. But on the other hand, my skeptical mind was challenged a lot by the data explained in the book, as my background was a scientific one with, let's say, a strong tendency for rationality.

From this tension between skepticism and gut arose in me a question: what was I going do with this book that was challenging my beliefs?

I still feel grateful I was open enough and even if I was far from being fully comfortable with all the data, I considered it as a theory I should test to see how valid it was.

Almost ten years later, I've been trained by the Institute and have tested during numerous hours the techniques on myself and on colleagues. I have now gained more experience and understanding about their subcellular psychobiology paradigm, but I'm still surprised by how much time, repetition and experiment I had to do to integrate the different techniques and start to feel more comfortable with them.

What is more surprising is the fact that this research also allowed them to work on what could be done to improve psychological health and well-being in a person. For example, work about peaks states lead to the discovery of what ISPS call "developmental events", events that when fully healed bring to the person a permanent state of happiness, peace…

Limitations with existing voice-hearing treatments

My clinical practice in psychiatry allows me to improve my knowledge in psychology and psychopathology. My job also gives me the chance to work with patients with different kinds of issues and I use different standard tools of psychotherapy, whether psychodynamics, cognitive behavioral therapy or EMDR

I've seen many patients who have been hearing voices for years despite unsuccessfully trying various treatments to stop them. I remember, in the beginning of my psychiatric studies, a woman who had been struggling with auditory hallucination for years. In the beginning, the voices were gentle and she was accustomed to them, but after a crisis the voices started to be aggressive. They were criticizing and commenting her behavior, making it very difficult to handle daily life with her husband and child. Treatment was difficult as she was very suspicious with voices that were telling her that people wanted to hurt her.

It is common belief that hearing voices is associated with psychosis, and it's partially true, with an estimated 74% of people suffering from schizophrenia that hear voices. But psychiatric research suggests that it is much more common as it is present in lots of other disorders like severe depression, PTSD, or even in the general population. An analysis of about 70 survey in 9 countries made by Beavan in 2011 suggested that around 5 to 15% of the population will hear voices. This fact is interesting as it allows us to decrease the stigma around voice hearing and make a move towards the ISPS understanding of voices that you will discover in this book.

Research on new treatments for voices

To give you a taste about how the process about voices described in the last chapter was developed, I will speak about my own experience with ISPS research. In 2014, I started to be involved in a new process that would impact the hearing voices problem. The hypothesis was that healing the right trauma in the proper developmental event would get rid of voices and some other symptoms. Over the years, I tested different processes that were invented by the main research team. Two adjectives perfectly describe my experiences while doing this: deep excitement, to test new processes and find a technique that would be working, and frustration, as I often wasn't able to finish the process or the changes were not stable.

To describe this research work, the metaphor of a puzzle seems pretty accurate to me. Imagine that you have the goal of finding a technique that can heal a symptom, in this case the main causes of auditory hallucinations. With all the experiments you made through the years, you have gained knowledge about the causes of this symptom, you guess which developmental event to work on and what traumas you need to heal in this event. Here you have a blurred view of the piece of the puzzle that are necessary to complete a working technique.

You start to put the pieces together while healing yourself in this event and it allows you see more clearly the trauma present in the developmental event, providing a more global view of the puzzle. While continuing healing you can't complete the puzzle as you sense you are not able to completely heal the event or the healing is not stable. You then know there is a part missing in your puzzle and you need to figure out what it is. The next step is to use this new information in developing and testing a new process that integrates this missing piece.

This research work allowed me to feel how much time, pain and effort it takes to arrive at a working technique in this field. I'm deeply grateful for all the work the ISPS members and volunteers made over the years to create all the techniques that can now be used safely and easily.

Technique validity

A logical question now is what is proven, or as we say in the medical field, is this data evidence-based? A few observations may help address this question:

In the field of therapy, there are lots of other techniques that can help people, but the map that has been pragmatically built by the ISPS during the last 30 years has one main advantage: it is based on experiments with the one goal of finding techniques that work, as seen from the client perspective of "I had a symptom - did it permanently disappear?" Over the years, this allowed them to find techniques that work on different symptoms (trauma/ voices/ anxiety...) and to gain understanding about the underlying causes.

A basic ISPS technique is working with trauma. An obvious example of trauma is Post Traumatic Stress Disorder (PTSD) where people that have gone through a very painful event continue to experience it, sometimes years after it happened, with repetition of mental images or emotions. One ISPS technique that works with those kinds of symptoms has similarities with EMDR in that it identifies the trauma(s) that causes the present symptom and then goes through a protocol to heal it. (The level of proof about EMDR in the scientific medical database is high and EMDR is one of the two specific techniques that are recommended by the WHO in the treatment of PTSD.)

But what about the other techniques that are described in this book? Some of them, like the body association or the silent mind technique, were developed by the institute years before and have been effective on many people.

The new experimental process I was writing about previously is still being researched and has been tested on far less people. So, for now, the level of proof on this is based on case reports.

I hope that in the future all this work will be evidence-based, and will become accessible to the largest number of people.

Thomas Gagey, MD
Yverdon les Bains, Switzerland
July 7, 2017

Acknowledgements

This project has spanned 22 years, with many, many people contributing their time, efforts and ideas. I want to acknowledge my many colleagues, students, and clients who volunteered to test our slowly evolving models and techniques. The friends and colleagues that were directly involved with this side project on voices follow in roughly chronological order:

Sheelo Bohm and Ron Mied for their training in regression during the early years of this work. And as always, thanks Sheelo for saving my life!

Dr. Ben Tong, my abnormal psychology professor and Ph.D. program mentor at the California Institute for Integral Studies; I so appreciated you personal encouragement over the years since I was your student.

John Heinegg and Paula Courteau on beautiful Hornby Island BC for the 15 years they've hung out with me, devoting their time and effort on this and other projects. And thanks Paula for all your editing of the many books we've done!

Gina Chick for her enthusiasm, time and efforts in testing new processes in 2006.

Matt Fox, for his pioneering work on body association techniques.

Thanks to all the staff of the Scottish Schizophrenia Clinic for your time, enthusiasm, and efforts. We may have failed back in 2008, but our combined efforts paved the way for later success.

Tony Clarkson, founder of the Sanctuary of Healing in the UK, whose financial donation helped keep us going during the difficult financial downturn of 2008-9.

Chant and Susanna Thomas, whose steadfast friendship and faith in me over the decades has kept me moving forward. Those months at your farm in 2010 and 2016 made all the difference.

Dr. Art McCarley, my colleague at Cal Poly, whose suggestions and friendship over the years has been invaluable. And to my cousins Ian and Merina Harriman of Nelson BC, whose steadfast encouragement has been a wonderful gift.

Liz and Mark Jory, my wonderful artist landlords in whose beautiful cabin on the water on Hornby Island I wrote the first draft of this book.

Frank Downey, my uncle, friend, and colleague in these adventures for so many years. And to Kimberly Braun, who worked with our staff in 2010-11 and encouraged me to get this material out into the world. And to Shayne McKenzie, our volunteer CEO since 2015, for encouraging us all, and for taking on this tough job of bringing our work to those who need it.

And thanks to my colleagues who volunteered their time to review this text: Sean Chiddy, Samsara Salier, Nemi Nath, Nicolai Hassing, Georg Parlow, Dr. Kirsten Lykkegaard, Dr. Maarten Willemsen, Dr. Thomas Gagey, and Dr. Mary Pellicer.

Finally, my very special thanks to my dear friends and colleagues Steve and Jessie Hsu, who encouraged me when times got tough, and whose generous donation made writing this book possible.

This work on voices was just a tiny part of the entire research project we were doing into subcellular psychobiology and prenatal developmental biology. The work by my colleagues to discover and understand this underlying biology is what made progress in the area of hearing voices possible. Thank you, all my many colleagues at the Institute for the Study of Peak States who have participated in this huge project of finding and exploring this new field.

About the illustrations and cover art

I also want to thank our staff researcher and graphic artist Piotr Kawecki of Poland for his beautiful cover art and several of the text figures. And I would also like to thank the Peak States certified therapist Lorenza Meneghini of Italy for her wonderful drawings that made the text more understandable and interesting.

Introduction

This book is about a fundamental discovery that links the terrible problem of schizophrenic voices to subcellular biology in a new and completely unsuspected way.

It's also about how most of our ordinary, everyday thoughts are also symptoms of the same underlying disease process, a species-wide fungal infection that affects nearly everyone alive. And how this disease has other severe and devastating psychological effects, such as the phenomena of dysfunctional cultural norms and cross-cultural aggression.

These pages tell a 22-year long story of discovery, disappointment, setbacks, and triumphs as we worked to solve this baffling problem. It is also the story of countless volunteer hours of suffering and frustration spent by dedicated, altruistic colleagues as they experimenting on themselves, trying to understand the cause of this problem and develop treatments.

We had several goals in mind when we wrote this book. First is the obvious one, ways to treat hearing voices. But we also hope that this book will introduce to the general public, clinicians, and academics our discoveries of a subcellular and developmental biology approach using quasi-psychological tools that can eliminate symptoms *and* be used to eliminate diseases as well. We earnestly hope that others will be inspired to use this to find new ways to treat diseases that current technologies cannot help.

This book is also just a small look into a much larger picture during those years, as we simultaneously worked to explore and comprehend the entirely new field of subcellular psychobiology. We hope you will enjoy this brief taste of what breakthrough research is really like.

Who is this book for?

Like a detective mystery, we deliberately wrote this book in a chronological story-like way so that anyone could follow along as we slowly unraveled the enigma of this disease. We did this step-by-step approach so that the startling conclusions we came to would make sense – otherwise, if we just summarized our results, it would be far too easy to simply dismiss our findings and stay with one's current beliefs. Thus, this book is for laypeople, therapists, and academics, with hopefully enough human-interest stories to make the academic content still fun to read.

We want this book to be empowering for people suffering from the hearing voices problem. We also want it to help the families of loved ones who suffer from this disease, either by helping them understand that there might be help, or by helping them understand that the problem is not some kind of tragic genetic, incurable defect in their loved one. After all, as you will see it turns out that they're just suffering from a fungal disease like the common athlete's foot fungus, albeit one harder to get rid of and much nastier in its effects.

This book is also used as an introductory textbook for a short course on training therapists in how to recognize and treat ribosomal voices and their associated problems. Detailed steps on how to make a person immune to the underlying causal disease have been omitted but are covered with handouts in class. However, the theory behind those treatments is covered in this book.

Thus, this book is designed for:
- Anyone who hears voices.
- Therapists and support people who want to help voice hearers.
- People who want a silent mind.
- Patients who have schizophrenia.
- Therapists who just want to know about new ways to help their clients.
- Those who want to learn more about subcellular psychobiology.
- Those who want to understand the latest breakthroughs in psycho-immunology.
- People interested in peak states (in particular the 'Listening to Silence' state).
- Mediators working with cross-cultural conflicts.
- Therapists working with multi-cultural adjustment problems.
- Therapists or laypeople who need a textbook for a short course in treating these diseases.

This book is *not* intended to be a full course for academics; rather, it is designed to be an introduction so that they would know that there is something new to learn. For details on subcellular and developmental psychobiology, we refer you to our other textbooks.

The stigma of 'hearing voices'

One of the biggest problems that people who hear voices face is the belief that they are mentally ill. In this book, we show that ribosomal voices, the most common form of voices, are caused by a subcellular fungal infection that has *nothing* to do with any hypothesized defect or flaw in their minds.

For decades the evidence that people who are 'hearing voices' are not usually mental ill has been accumulating in academic journals, and by the public outreach efforts of Intervoice and the Hearing Voices Network. However, this evidence has been ignored, discounted, or rejected by research organizations and health authorities around the world. Instead, most continue to assume that voices show an intrinsic disorder that only drugs can help control, in spite of their side effects, temporary nature, and lack of effectiveness for many people.

We believe that one of the biggest reasons for keeping this 'status quo' is because there has been no clear biological model that could explain the voices. Hence, this book was written to give just such an explanation so that the entire field can move forward. But it is not enough to just say that an interaction of trauma with a subcellular fungal parasite can make voices. We back this up with simple treatments based on this model that actually work, demonstrating that this model has validity. Once other researchers understand what they are trying to accomplish, we expect that they will find new ways to treat this disease, perhaps with an antifungal drug.

Introducing the new field of subcellular psychobiology

This book also has another goal – to bring the entirely new field of subcellular psychobiology to people's awareness. We do this by introducing, step by step, some of the breakthroughs that led to our discovery of this new field. And then we demonstrate how treatments based on this actually work on one of the worst and most baffling mental disorders in the world – schizophrenia.

This subcellular psychobiology approach allows researchers to link psychological symptoms to the underlying subcellular diseases that indirectly cause them. Up until now no one even suspected that they should be looking *inside* the cell for the cause of these 'psychological' or 'mental' disorders. More importantly, it shows how psychological techniques can be used to rapidly and permanently eliminate symptoms caused by these problems.

The implications are profound. This introduces an entirely new way of understanding and treating disease. The ribosomal voices in this book are just *one* of many mental disorders that can be understood using subcellular psychobiology. By demonstrating that it can be used to understand and help treat aspects of one of the biggest problems in mental health, we hope this will spur interest in finding the causes and new treatments for *other* mental health disorders.

As in any branch of science, once a problem is identified and understood, and a technique identified that can demonstrate the model, other ways of solving the problem will be found. There are a lot of brilliant people out there who can take whatever mental health disorder they're working on and find new solutions. Our hope is that this book will point them in the right direction with a model that explains these heretofore mysterious and tragic problems.

A breakthrough in psycho-immunology

There is another key breakthrough that this book demonstrates. After we isolated a fungal cause for ribosomal voices, we came up with a *psychological* treatment that reliably makes people completely immune to this disease. This has stunning implications that may not be obvious – this approach can work with *any* disease, not just ones involving mental disorders.

In past decades there was a lot of interest in the idea that psychological approaches might be able to cure physical diseases. In spite of some truly astonishing individual successes, no consistently reliable techniques were developed, and so for the most part interest and efforts to create more effective 'psycho-immunology' (later called psychoneuroimmunlogy) techniques had faded away.

In this book we demonstrate that this is actually possible to make people immune to a fungus by using quasi-psychological techniques that interact with *subcellular* processes, prenatal developmental stages, and epigenetic damage - something that no one realized was even relevant or possible to do. Unfortunately, with the current state of the art, each disease needs individual investigation and a new treatment. We hope this spurs development of even better techniques from other researchers. But in the years to come, we expect an entire *class* of diseases (bacterial, fungal, viral, or prion) can be treated all at once with this approach.

Again, we hope the publication of this book will spur interest in applying these sorts of psychological techniques to other diseases. In these days of increasing resistance to antibiotics, of endemic diseases in third world countries that no one has funds to treat, it makes sense to explore treatment modalities that are not only permanent but virtually free in comparison to standard drug treatments (ignoring the relatively inexpensive research costs). After all, some of these techniques can be shown on a

YouTube video, with patients simply following the steps, as if doing yoga poses or repairing a car.

The limitations of this book, liability, and safety issues

This book is intended for *educational* purposes only. That means we *only* recommend you work with a therapist who has been trained in this material. These techniques are fast, and if you work with a therapist who charges for results, it is an inexpensive way to get the best possible outcome. This is exactly like taking your taxes to a professional. It doesn't cost that much, they know exactly what to do, and you don't need to learn the constantly changing tax codes. If you don't know a therapist who can help, go online and find a therapist certified by the Institute for the Study of Peak States – or talk your favorite health professional into getting the training.

Secondly, we certainly *don't* recommend that you start experimenting on yourself! Research in this area is potentially dangerous – it takes us years of testing before a technique or process is ready for clients. Don't become a human guinea pig! Let trained and experienced professionals who know a lot more about all this find any risks or problems.

Third, the processes in this book are *not* a fix for all schizophrenics. The treatments for ribosomal voices in this book help only a relatively small proportion of the severely mentally ill schizophrenic population (although it does work for most of the 'hearing voices' population we've treated). Nor does it address the entire range of possible 'voice hearing' problems. There are other, much less common diseases that can cause similar symptoms. In the last chapter of this book we look at some of these problems and their differential diagnosis.

Lastly, if you are a therapist treating this client group, we refer you to the *Subcellular Psychobiology Diagnosis Handbook* for specific diagnostic criteria for the material in this book (as well as for many other subcellular problems).

Trademarks and 'pay for results'

We have several trademarks for the work we do. Both Whole-Hearted Healing and Peak States are registered trademarks around the world, and both the Silent Mind Technique (which is actually a collection of processes for making the mind silent) and the Body Association Technique are also trademarked. But why?

The answer is quality control. As other technique developers have found to their dismay, once a technique is published and becomes popular, unscrupulous people will advertise that they either teach or use the techniques to attract business. (This problem shows up in virtually every business, not just in psychology.) The problem is that what they teach or do often has no resemblance to the original technique. EFT and NLP are both good examples of this kind of disaster. EMDR, on the other hand, is a good example of a trademarked technique where the label actually means something that everyone can agree on. But let's say someone does correctly teach the material in this book. What's the problem? Unfortunately with wide-ranging, cutting-edge techniques like these, there is still a lot of material that is not yet published, so trying to teach without this knowledge can potentially cause safety issues. Worse, these people simply don't have the practical experience that they need in order to teach adequately.

Secondly, as techniques evolve, you want to know about any improvements or any new problems discovered. An organization that holds the trademark has incentive to do this, while others who are merely copying (or worse, making stuff up) will simply ignore any revisions or improvements. We've actually seen this when our material was translated into other languages – the people doing it were not interested in keeping up to date with new material, because they were only focused on income, not quality.

Finally, therapists licensed by our Institute also agree to a 'pay for results' with their clients. Working with therapists who adhere to this kind of quality standard is a huge, huge advantage that other's can't or won't offer. So, if you are a consumer, why not look for therapists who offer this?

Where can I learn more?

We keep our research results and course offerings updated online at www.PeakStates.com. (For example, we offer a training course on the material in this book.) We also publish textbooks that can be purchased internationally and in several languages through Amazon or your local bookstore.

Our 2014 *Subcellular Psychobiology Diagnosis Handbook* is the first book in this series on Peak States® Therapy. That book identifies a number of subcellular damages and diseases that cause symptoms in people. However, unlike this book, it was written for practicing therapists that needed a desk reference for diagnosing and treating clients. If you are a therapist and want more specific guidance on differential diagnosis and symptoms of the material in this book, we refer you there. If you are a layperson I would suggest saving your money and just read the free first two summary chapters on Amazon.

If you are a therapist or a layperson interested in helping clients or in self-help, and want to know about regression therapy or subcellular psychobiology techniques, we refer you to *The Whole-Hearted Healing™ Workbook* (2013) by Paula Courteau, and *The Basic Whole-Hearted Healing™ Manual* (2004) by Grant McFetridge Ph.D. and Mary Pellicer M.D. We suggest starting with Paula's book – it is better written, has newer techniques, and is designed for self-help.

If you are a layperson or an academic interested in our discoveries in positive psychology and peak states of consciousness, trauma, prenatal regression, prenatal developmental events, and the primary cell, we refer you to *Peak States of Consciousness* volumes 1 (2004), 2 (2008) and 3 (not yet published). If you are a layperson, we suggest starting with volume 1. The follow-on Volume 2 is much more detailed and written primarily for professionals in this field.

In the near future, we plan to publish more in this series of books, each focused on specific areas (addictions, suicide, spiritual emergencies, etc.) that use our approach for treatment. We do this because they offer totally new ways to understand and heal these formally intractable diseases and disorders.

Grant McFetridge, Ph.D.
Institute for the Study of Peak States
Hornby Island, BC Canada

Section 1

A Slow Journey of Discovery

Chapter 1

Setting the Stage

When I sat down to write this book, I realized that just some dry recital of biological facts would not help people accept or use our discoveries. My colleagues and I had made fundamental breakthroughs; but real breakthroughs are usually uncomfortable and all too easily rejected without trial or consideration, as has been seen over and over in the history of science. So instead, in the next few chapters I'll lead you through, step by step, the trail we blazed that spans over thirty years of successes, failures, and unexpected discoveries. Like any detective mystery, I hope you will follow along, thinking about the clues we found and the experiments we ran, as we derived this entirely new way of understanding the causes of mental illness.

But how does something like this even get started? And why did we go in a direction that no one ever imagined could lead to completely new, unsuspected biology?

To help answer this question, in this chapter I'll start by sharing a bit of my own story. It's one of tragedy, unexpected twists and turns, and friendships with a number of remarkable individuals who encouraged or taught me during those early years. It's also about an unusual combination of multi-disciplinary experiences and a singular motivation that led me off the beaten track and made these breakthroughs possible.

Tragedy Strikes

I was eight years old when our family tragedy started.

My father, an M.D. in internal medicine, was employed as a researcher for a pharmaceutical company in Canada. When I was in third grade, he took a new research job and so we moved to upstate New York, to a small quiet town called Croton-on-the-Hudson. Our house was at the end of a road in a beautiful hardwood forest, with a small pond that had turtles and muskrats. My younger brother Scott and I loved that place, and we had wonderful adventures exploring that forest.

I was in third grade when dad was admitted to the local hospital and misdiagnosed with a mental disorder. Mom, who was a nurse, while visiting him spotted that his appendix had ruptured and he was actually dying. (Rarely, some schizophrenics have blunting of pain, although it usually occurs late in the course of the disease.) Eventually dad returned home, with tubes still in his belly as the raging infection was brought under control. For many months he remained at home recovering. But he was not the same afterwards. He would retreat into dark places in the house, and started to become unreasonably angry towards my mom, something completely out of character for this normally very kind and gentle man.

Over the following years dad's mental condition continued to deteriorate. He would slowly worsen, then slowly recover, with each cycle more severe than the last. My mom truly loved him, and it was heartbreaking for her. But love was not enough – it could not stop his descent into madness. Eventually, mom was forced to recognize that nothing she could do could help. At that point, dad could no longer work, or even communicate, so her brother Frank took him in during one of his worse episodes, and mom went to the University of British Columbia to finish her nursing degree, so she could get work to support her children and herself.

There was a kind of tacit agreement in the family to not talk about dad's schizophrenia during those childhood years. Looking back, my brother and I wish we had been more open with each other about what was happening and how we felt. Sadly, we missed the opportunity to support and help each other in the face of this terrible pain.

With the support of some of his closest friends, dad was able to continue to work for the next few decades. He even came to my wedding when I was 24. But eventually, his condition deteriorated to the point where he was admitted into an extended care facility in Alberta, and he never left it again until his death. During my thirties and forties, my brother, sister and I would make yearly pilgrimages, week-long trips up to visit him, but each year his condition was worse, until finally he was barely able to move or communicate. I did not really want to make those trips, as the father I had known as a child and young man was almost entirely gone. I felt a sense of family obligation, but this stranger who had been my father in truth somewhat repelled me.

Walking in Beauty

At this point, we're going to take a detour so you can get an understanding of how I, who did not want anything to do with mental illness, ended up working on schizophrenia. It turns out to be very relevant to finding a solution to this problem, as it caused me to take a totally new and unique direction.

My childhood was a study in contrasts. On the one hand, my father had schizophrenia. On the other hand, my mom and most of her extended family were unusually mentally healthy. But theirs was not just a matter of degree; rather, they experienced life in a fundamentally different and more positive way than most people could even imagine. And my sister and I were also blessed to have gotten whatever it was. But since we had been born with it, it just seemed normal and, like a fish in water, we did not really recognize it consciously. It was just the way most of our extended family was.

By high school, I was really starting to notice that my friends and acquaintances simply did not react to life as I did. These differences were becoming more and more apparent as I got older. When I was 15, I was very fortunate to get a summer job working at the Boy Scout Camp Omache, and for the first time in my life I met, not only one, but three others like myself. I was thrilled to realize that this was not only something that could be found in people outside of my extended family, it was something in its own right, a distinct way of being. Better, these staff members showed me it was possible to temporarily induce whatever it was that we had into many of our campers using song, enthusiasm and wilderness experiences. This was when I found out what I truly wanted to do with my life – to be able to give our amazing state of being permanently to others. But as I assumed that what we had must be genetic, I put that dream aside and went on with my life.

More background: aliveness - the Walking in Beauty state
Surprisingly, none of the teachers from the many spiritual paths that I knew of had ever heard of this fundamentally important state of being. Eventually I met Dr. Tom Pinkson, who immediately recognized it from First Nations traditions, where it is sometimes referred to as 'Walking in Beauty', or 'the Beauty Way'. I also found one psychology author, Dr. Harville Hendrix, who aptly called it 'aliveness'. The state is characterized by a feeling that one is filled with a feeling of life, and the world also radiates a sense of life. There is no unconscious underlying fear in a person, and one does what one feels is the right thing to do by referring to oneself rather than to the guidance of others. Spiritual truths are obvious, so much so one wonders why people talk about them. To an outside observer, the state is noticeable because a person in it simply doesn't normally experience or get triggered by traumatic feelings,

no matter what the cause. (This aspect of the state is called 'invulnerability' or 'resilience' in the psychological literature.)

A Career in Electrical Engineering

How did growing up with a mentally ill father affect my life and career?

Well, you might imagine that it made me want to become an MD like dad so I could find a cure for his disease. However, nothing could be further from the truth. Instead, I wanted to get as far away from sick people as I could. I believed, like most people at the time, that his mental disorder was an inherited genetic problem and hence hopeless to really cure. This also made me decide to never have any children so I would not pass on any of his defective genes to them. I was pretty sure that I would not get mentally ill like my dad, as I could find no trace of his symptoms in myself, but I was not going to rule that possibility out.

After high school, I went to university to become an electrical engineer. Like Steve Jobs of Apple Computers, I felt that this field was going to be the way to really make a difference to the world. Although it was not possible to see this at the time, this career choice would prove invaluable later, giving me tools and an engineer's orientation towards solving problems that I could never have gotten any other way.

After four years of working as a research and design engineer for the Hewlett Packard company, I felt strongly that I wanted to teach at the university level so I could also interact and make a difference in other's lives directly. I was fortunate to be admitted to Stanford University; being there was probably the most fun I've ever had, like drinking knowledge from a fire hose. Sadly, my wife did not like the academic environment, and after my Master's in electrical engineering was finished, we left and I went back into research and development. We divorced soon after, but by that time my life's course had been derailed.

Thus, by my mid-thirties, I was a successful research and development engineer, consultant, and occasional university lecturer. Even more importantly, I'd had over a decade's experience in cutting-edge research and development. I'd been apprenticed long enough, working for some of the best in the field, to have become competent in my craft. As an example, at the very first minute of my very first day as a lecturer at Cal Poly, a student stood up at the beginning of class and angrily asked me "why do you think you can teach us anything?" Apparently he had become very frustrated by some of his other professors. Fortunately, by this time I really was an expert in my field, so I smiled calmly at him and proceeded to explain my background. That first class and I had a great time as I started to learn this new skill of teaching. And it was just as much fun as I had hoped when I made that move to Stanford years ago! (Over a decade later, it also gave me the confidence and skill to start teaching experimental, immersive trauma therapy courses - a key step in moving my early explorations forward.)

Research using a multi-disciplinary approach

I want to stress that those years spent to master research and development skills in engineering were invaluable to my work later in a completely different field, working on the biology of schizophrenia. True, the specifics were different, and I rarely again used my math skills, but the way of creating models, deriving testable experiments, and having a sense of how multiple variable simultaneously interact would be absolutely vital to our project. And in both psychology and electrical engineering, I could not taste, touch or smell what I was working on. Instead, because I was always at the edge of what was possible with current technology, I generally had to think up testable implications and create a prototype measurement tool to try and observe the subtle operations of my latest cutting-edge trial circuit (or psychological process); then think up more tools and tests to measure the other tools to see if they were actually working properly. Oddly enough, electrical engineering research and psychological research were virtually the same in that respect. And both required the ability to create very good models – you had to be able to predict what would happen if you did such and so, in order to test that you really understood what was going on. And both engineering and psychology research took a tremendous tolerance for frustration and setbacks.

Probably the biggest hurdle I found later in psychological and biological research was in finding colleagues who shared at least some of that engineering problem solving skill set. Without it, they were generally unable to understand and accept the process of research, where nothing goes in a straight line or on schedule. With some notable exceptions, over the years I found that it was generally better to take an engineer with research and development experience and train them in the relevant biology, rather than trying to train a biologist, doctor or therapist in how to do breakthrough research. The mindsets were, for most people, just too fundamentally different.

Shifting to Psychology

During my divorce when I was 29, I suddenly lost my life-long Beauty Way state. Although it felt like I'd suddenly been sent to hell, it was also an incredibly exciting time for me, because this loss meant that that state must not be genetic in origin. After all, if it had been a genetic DNA sequence then I could never have lost it. So my childhood ambition of giving this state to others was now a real possibility. But how?

I started to seriously explore that childhood passion while continuing on with my engineering career. This was 1985 and I was living in California, so as you might imagine there was a whole potpourri of spiritual traditions, psychological approaches and a number of other unusual beliefs to investigate. To get a better understanding of what the psychological field knew about this topic, in 1992 I also enrolled in a psychology Ph.D. program at what many considered the foremost transpersonal psychology school at the time, the California Institute for Integral Studies. I had the great good luck to have gotten Professor Ben Tong who specialized in abnormal psychology as my mentor during those years.

Then I started to get sick.

I had some mysterious illness that was causing me to lose weight. I worked with a number of doctors and, as you might imagine, I also tried all sorts of alternative cures (remember, I was living in California in the 80s), all without success. Over the course of a year, I came to look like a starving refugee, just skin over bones. Eventually I could barely walk, and finally my latest physician told me to get my affairs in order as I had only about three weeks left to live.

The next day, while slowly walking into the local post office, I ran into an old friend, Sheelo Bohm. He took one look at me and said "You don't look so good!" So I explained to him about my illness and prognosis, he scratched his chin and said, "You work with me three times and I'll save your life." As we'd been friends who meditated together at the Ring of Bone Zendo, I knew he worked as a cutting edge therapist. And sure enough, on our third session, using a modified form of Grof's Holotropic Breathwork, we cracked the cause of my illness. It turned out that I was dying because I felt huge despair that I could never have what I really wanted in life, to see other people living in amazing states of being. And so I had unconsciously decided that there was no point in living anymore. When we finally uncovered it, I grieved for about thirty minutes, and then I just knew I would be well. I knew that this, something that was completely outside my conscious awareness, was what had been killing me.

This story is relevant because of what happened next.

Over the next few months, I was ecstatic to have survived. As I reflected on what had happened, I started to really think about trauma. During those years, most experts did not consider trauma of much importance to people's lives, except for the problem of PTSD (post traumatic stress disorder) in war veterans, which was assumed to be incurable. But after my experience of nearly dying, it was clear that unconscious trauma could have a much more serious effect than I had ever suspected.

I eventually realized that at this point in my life, I wanted to try to figure out some way to eliminate all traumas from my psyche. After all, what other completely unrecognized land mines might still be buried in my subconscious?

Developing a Regression Technique

Unfortunately, during most of those years I didn't know of any really effective trauma healing technique. True, there were a number of bodywork and breathing approaches, but nothing you could just point at an issue to heal it. However, behind the scenes the whole new field of trauma therapy was starting to happen, cumulating in the groundbreaking 1996 article in the Family Therapy Networker on PTSD (Post Traumatic Stress Disorder) treatment therapies that actually worked. Up to that point, it was assumed that trauma was simply incurable.

More background: trauma technique breakthroughs
Trauma can be defined as an emotionally painful, stuck memory that simply won't stop hurting without intervention. The key trauma-healing treatments, EMDR (Eye Movement Desensitization and Reprocessing), TIR (Traumatic Incident Reduction), and TFT (Thought Field Therapy) were developed in the 1980s and 1990s. Just as importantly from my perspective, groundbreaking work was also being done in the area of prenatal and perinatal trauma. Authors like Stanislav Grof MD, Dr. Arthur Janov, Graham Farrant MD, and people in organizations like the Association for Pre- and Perinatal Psychology were making discoveries that were tying prenatal trauma to life-long physical and emotional problems.

And both the humanistic and transpersonal psychology movements were taking a good look at a plethora of spiritual and mystical experiences that had been ignored up to that time. One example was the publication of Dr. Grof's groundbreaking book on spiritual emergencies in 1989, as it suddenly put a lot of these phenomena into an understandable framework.

So, my next order of business was to figure out a simple, reliable method to heal trauma. And not just any trauma - I wanted to be able to also target prenatal trauma. More than that, I wanted an investigative tool, as my intuition was telling me that prenatal trauma was key to understanding why some people had exceptional states of consciousness while most did not.

Fortunately, I had already encountered something I thought might help. About six months earlier, I had met a therapist named Ron Mied at a conference on shamanism. As we'd sat outside chatting during lunch, I found his skeptical but practical attitude mirrored my own. And he had already made a key discovery about the nature of trauma. He had realized that all traumas were frozen moments in time, but from an external, out-of-body viewpoint, exactly like watching a freeze-frame image on TV. In the spring of 1994, and over the next year or so I apprenticed myself to both Ron and to Sheelo, working with them to explore and master their techniques.

Unfortunately, I didn't find that their methods met my goals, so I took their insights and my own ideas and experiences, and ended up developing a somewhat different approach to healing trauma. My new technique also had another tremendous advantage – I could use it to easily access pre-birth experiences in order to study them. Over the next seven years or so I continued to refine my approach, working with thousands of clients, testing, improving, and exploring completely unknown pre- and perinatal developmental events. This became the Whole-Hearted Healing regression technique for trauma healing.

The stage is now set. In the next chapter we'll see how the first discovery about schizophrenia was made.

Key Points

- In the last 25 years, effective techniques to heal trauma and PTSD (Post Traumatic Stress Disorder) have become available. These include EMDR, EFT, and a host of others.
- By using appropriate techniques, people can relive their own prenatal and perinatal traumas.
- The field of prenatal and perinatal psychology describes experiences that are not generally known by laypeople.
- The Whole-Hearted Healing regression technique for trauma healing was specifically developed to investigate prenatal events.
- Some people are born with unusually positive, continuous 'peak' states of being.

Suggested Reading

On trauma healing:

- *EMDR: The Breakthrough Therapy for Overcoming Anxiety, Stress, and Trauma* (1998), by Francis Shapiro and Margot Forrest.
- *The EFT Manual* (2011), by Gary Craig.

- "Going for the Cure" (July/August 1996), *Family Therapy Networker*, By M. S. Wylie, 20(4) pgs. 20-37.
- *Traumatic Incident Reduction* (1999), by Gerald French and Chrys Harris.

On regression techniques:
- *Regression Therapy: A Handbook for Professionals*, Vol. 1 and 2 (1993), Winafred Blake Lucas.
- *The Basic Whole-Hearted Healing™ Manual*, 3rd Ed. (2004), by Grant McFetridge Ph.D. and Mary Pellicer, M.D.
- *The Whole-Hearted Healing Workbook* (2013), by Paula Courteau.

On peak states of consciousness:
- *Peak States of Consciousness: Theory and Applications*, Volumes 1 (2004) and 2 (2008), by Grant McFetridge Ph.D., Jacquelyn Aldana, and James Hardt Ph.D.
- *Peak States of Consciousness: Theory and Applications*, Volume 2 (2008), by Grant McFetridge Ph.D. and Wes Geitz.
- *The Adventure of Self Discovery* (1988), by Stanislav Grof M.D.

Chapter 2

The First Breakthrough

This chapter explores the first breakthrough that made a connection between prenatal trauma, everyday thoughts in the mind, and schizophrenic 'voices'.

This account is a good example of how cutting-edge research really works; trying to attain one goal can sometimes lead to the completely unexpected. I was not investigating schizophrenia at all; I was trying to derive a more inclusive model of the psyche to help with my work on exceptional 'peak' states of consciousness. But it was investigating the enigmatic phenomena of channeling, demonic possession and 'entities' from this lens that actually led to a first treatment for schizophrenic voices.

This breakthrough answered a lot of puzzling questions. It turns out that virtually *all* people have this same problem, whether you call it mind chatter, obsessive thoughts, disembodied spirits, channeling, possession, or voices. The only difference is one's ability to mute the volume of the words. It is a two-stage disorder – the first, where the voices are in the background and considered to be a normal part of life; the second, when trauma triggers a lack of suppression and the voices become intrusively loud. (In later chapters we'll see there can be other factors, but this statement holds true for most people.)

I'll end this chapter with the story of one of the most important moments in my life – curing my own father of schizophrenia.

Making a model that covers all of psychology

During the 1990s, I lived in a small one-room cabin in the foothills of the Sierras in California. I would occasionally work as an engineer, university lecturer, or even a physical laborer to pay the rent, but I was primarily focused on my research into prenatal experiences. I was slowly building up a model, a new understanding of how the psyche actually worked, one that could actually help me understand and heal people's issues.

In my clinical psychology doctoral program I'd been required to memorize over 30 different 'maps of the mind', but unfortunately I did not find any of them useful for helping people; nor could any of them cover all of the problems and experiences that people were having. After all, if a model is truly valid, it should be testable and useful in a variety of ways. So, like the engineer I was, I also started investigating other types of experiences that might also shed light on the psyche. To be valid, my model also had to include and explain all phenomena – not just culturally acceptable ones – such as near-death experiences, spiritual emergencies, past lives, shamanic healing, and so on.

When I began this project, I had a rather Rogerian viewpoint of the human condition, probably because it resonates with the Beauty Way state of being. Before I got deeply involved in my investigations, I tended to assume people's problems and beliefs simply stemmed from painful experiences in their lives. My worldview was quite socially acceptable, simple and straightforward. From my perspective now, thirty years later, I was very naïve. I simply was not yet exposed to the rich amount of other phenomena that were being explored by laypeople and professionals in the transpersonal and prenatal fields.

More background: Carl Rogers

The late Carl Rogers, founder of the humanistic psychology movement, revolutionized psychotherapy with his concept of "client-centered therapy." He based his life's work on his fundamental belief in the human potential for growth. His book *'A Way of Being'* is an excellent introduction.

As I started to look into various unusual 'spiritual' or 'psychic' experiences, it was becoming clear that people were dealing with them by actually holding two completely different worldviews in their minds. On the one hand, they would go see doctors if they were sick or injured. On the other hand, they treated these strange, unusual experiences as if they had their own set of rules, ones completely divorced from science or biology. As an engineer, I knew I needed something that would tie all these unusual experiences together with known biology and psychology.

I did not know it then, but unfortunately the information needed to generate a unified psychobiology model simply did not exist at the time. In the next chapter we'll see the breakthrough in 2002 that finally allowed us to link psychology to biology, and how that model eventually allowed us to understand the biological cause of schizophrenic voices. But for now, let's get back to looking at some of the relevant experiential data...

Channeling

When I was in California in the 1980s and early 1990s, there was a lot of interest in the phenomena of 'channeling' (also called spirit communication or mediumship). People were claiming that disembodied voices would tell them profound spiritual truths or give them important information to share. Some would go further than this, and assume another persona and speak as if they were another person.

More background: channeling
I highly recommend Arthur Hastings or John Klimo's books on the phenomenon of channeling, written back in the 80s. They both approached their investigation as open minded, objective scientists, something that was sorely lacking in most accounts at the time.

Given my interest in radical consciousness change, I was at least prepared to investigate the claims I was hearing. After all, in my regression work I'd already encountered phenomena that I would have sworn were just figments of people's overactive imagination, such as past life trauma, 'holes' in the body, and a host of others. (Yes, I had to 'eat crow' quite a number of times!) More, there were a lot of honest, smart professionals who I knew and respected who were also encountering phenomena that were completely outside of everyday beliefs. So, if channeling was actually possible (acknowledging that there were probably a number of frauds simply making money off this new fad), getting answers from a channel might be a fast way to find out how to induce the Beauty Way state into people. I'm a pretty practical engineer – if it actually turned out to be real, then maybe I could get some answers; and honestly, I was also just plain curious.

At the time I was living in Nevada City, California, a wonderful small mountain town that had an incredible number of highly creative and talented people. Conveniently, there was a lot of channeling going on, making it easy to gather data. Surprisingly, I soon found out that there were a lot of channelers who only wanted it to stop. And as I watched people who had another personality speak through them to give talks or answer questions, I also noticed another important piece of data. The longer they channeled in a session, the more distress their body was in. And I soon noticed that the content of the channeled 'messages' was not useful, and in fact was full of platitudes and untestable claims. For example, many people would ask channelers about painful feelings and situations in their lives - if these channelers were speaking from some greater level of being, why did none of them teach meridian tapping (EFT) or bilateral stimulation (EMDR) to eliminate trauma? Those simple techniques were one of the biggest breakthroughs ever in the field of healing and human development, but were not available until another decade had passed. Clearly, in spite of what people wanted to believe, channeling was not what people hoped it was.

So what, exactly, was really going on? And then I ran into something even stranger.

'Entities' and 'Demonic Possession'

Like most people of my generation who'd gotten the pants scared off them from the movie 'The Exorcist', I knew about possession and demonic entities. But aside from Hollywood horror movies, I assumed it was just a holdover of Christian beliefs from centuries ago. You can't imagine how surprised I was to actually encounter it for the first time.

Over the years, I would occasionally trigger this phenomenon in clients during regression healing, perhaps once in every three hundred sessions or so. Let me give you a couple of examples to illustrate the problem. In one case, I was at a conference about trauma therapies. During my demonstration of regression in front of about a dozen people, the client (a capable and mentally healthy therapist) went into a full-on demonic possession episode, just like in the movies. When this happens, a very disturbing feeling of evil radiates from the client, with a sense that you, the therapist, might become forever contaminated. It stopped when we finished healing the traumatic event that she'd regressed into. In another case, I was working with a close friend who was using a 'distant healing' technique on me when suddenly she started screaming in panic that something evil was in her body. It disappeared when I had her do simple meridian tapping on the feeling. (Interestingly, the next day this woman could no longer recall the incident, in spite of the fact that she'd been so terrified just the day before.)

At this point, I also started paying attention to people who talked about 'entities', evil or otherwise. In fact, I was running into self-styled healers who said they could look at a person and 'see' something that they interpreted as an entity inside or near the person. Of course, it was pretty clear that some of these healers were simply delusional, but others appeared both sane and competent.

Whatever this phenomenon was, it could be 'seen' by others. As an example of this, I recall a session where I was getting help healing a trauma via the phone when:

"Suddenly, my teacher who was on the phone across an ocean let out a scream and said he'd call back. Later, he said that at a particular point in my healing, he'd suddenly seen something leave me and race towards him. This blew him away, but he recovered none the worse for it eventually. A while later, I was speaking with a Hawaiian woman shaman, and she mentioned that I was 'possessed' by an 'entity'. And in fact, several people around this time mentioned it. It was quite embarrassing for me. Of course, at this point I couldn't 'see' what they were talking about, so like you I was a bit suspicious of it all. Yet, the indirect data kept mounting up..."

I also started to investigate the shamanic concepts of soul stealing and soul loss, figuring that perhaps these indigenous ideas were somehow related. After all, just because the Greeks believed that Zeus threw thunderbolts didn't mean that lightning wasn't real.

More background: shamanism
The 1970s through the 1990s were a time of interest in saving the rapidly disappearing indigenous knowledge of shamanism. Dr. Michael Harner's book *'The Way of the Shaman'* was excellent because of its worldwide scope and lack of dismissive Western cultural bias.

By this point, it was pretty clear that people talking about 'entities' and 'demonic possession' were describing real, consistent and widespread experiential phenomena, even if their *explanations* were based on pure imagination or pre-science worldviews. They were obviously *not* mentally ill, in spite of what they were describing. So what was really going on? Did it relate to schizophrenia? In the next section we'll get the first clue.

The first breakthrough

As I've said, my primary motivation was to find a way to give humanity exceptional states of being - but how?

Then I had an idea. I had been a Zen Buddhist meditator for a number of years by this point, and it occurred to me that perhaps, just perhaps, that mediation teachers' emphasis on quieting one's thoughts (the 'monkey mind' as it is sometimes called) might be a way into profound states. So I decided to explore this idea using my new approach to trauma healing and regression, but it wasn't obvious how to connect trauma to random thoughts in my mind as I meditated. I still had no interest in schizophrenia at this point, as I assumed the two phenomena were completely unrelated. Soon I'd find out differently.

In January of 1995 serendipity struck during a Holotropic breathwork session. I became aware of what felt like the invisible presence of a really angry, nasty old guy who was somehow stuck to me. It was pretty darn exciting, because now I had my very own 'entity' that I could experiment on.

At this point, you might wonder if I felt like I'd become mentally ill, but no – my everyday experience hadn't changed, and it was tough to even sense this thing. Also, I knew a lot of really capable therapists who had also encountered these in themselves or their clients and were also puzzled by it. There was a sense that all of us were working on the cutting edge, exploring something that had been recognized traditionally but ignored or misunderstood in our modern society.

I tried a few different ways to get rid of it, whatever it was, but didn't make any progress. Then I had the idea of hooking myself up to a GSR (galvanic skin response) meter to use it like a lie detector, to see if I could interrogate my own subconscious. And it worked. The meter would twitch whenever my associate would ask a question my body didn't want to answer. What we figured out was that my body wanted to keep that invisible angry old guy nearby, and wasn't about to let me get rid of him, but I had no idea why. I came out of that session pretty darn puzzled, thinking that I must have an insane body consciousness!

More background: the triune brain

Neuroscientist Dr. Paul MacLean of the US National Institute of Mental Health in the 1970s discovered that all primates have a 'triune' brain – with a body (reptilian or r-complex), heart (mammalian or limbic brain), and mind (primate or neocortex), each controlling different bodily functions.

Surprisingly, our work with regression led to the discovery that, from a psychological viewpoint, each triune brain is self-aware, each 'thinks' quite differently (with either body sensations, emotions, or thoughts), and they act like children as they compete with each other for attention or control. These awarenesses make up part of what is loosely called the subconscious.

A few weeks later, I was still puzzling over this. Then a breakthrough happened unexpectedly on February 26, 1995. That day I wrote in my journal:

"As I was working [on sawing a piece of plywood], I was thinking about my attraction to angry women, just as I had been talking to Lauri at lunch (about it). Then the thought passed through my mind, I think it was, that an entity surrounds me like an angry mom. And the idea that it was during birth that I was surrounded by an angry mom, probably feeling deserted by dad.

"Anyway, whatever the exact thought was, my chest *moved* and still feels kind of sore [from this insight experience]. I tried to start sawing again after a few minutes, but I was too blown away. So I just sat for about 15 minutes. 'Aftershocks' continue."

I expanded on that in a letter to a friend two weeks later:

"I was sawing a piece of plywood, working on why I was physically attracted to angry women (just two, but the second one indicated a bad pattern). With a flash, it all came together! I briefly relived a piece of the birth trauma, which knocked me on my butt for 15 minutes.

"It turns out that everyone's advice on this topic was bad, because they had not healed this in themselves! Very few healers I know have gone into the birth trauma, and the problem was located there. People's advice was to look at why I might be angry inside, and heal my own anger. Well, I really pursued that track, and got nowhere, entity-wise. It turns out that the real problem was completely different.

"During the birth process, my mom got really angry at my dad. As a fetus trying to survive in this hellish experience of birth, I made an association between survival and the sensation of the feeling of anger surrounding and penetrating me (that's how the body consciousness experiences the mother in the womb). This was a near match to having an angry entity in my body field. This was also why I was attracted to angry women, a manifestation of the same experience. So I couldn't give up the entity because it felt like my survival was at stake."

It was an amazing sensation as key pieces of the puzzle fell into place in that one moment. What I'd done was connect the experience of having 'entities' to prenatal trauma. In particular, I was trying to get mom to protect and save me from being hurt, somewhat similar to a drowning kid reaching out to their mother. The feeling that my survival was at stake was now *associated* with mom's emotional tone. Over the next few days, the rest of the pieces quickly fell into place. And I quickly realized that my annoying, intrusive thoughts during meditation were actually coming from different fixed locations in space around me, each with a characteristic emotional tone. Aha! This tied the idea of ordinary, everyday mind chatter to the experience of 'entities' ('voices'). Each stream of thoughts has its own emotional tone, verbal content, and location in space.

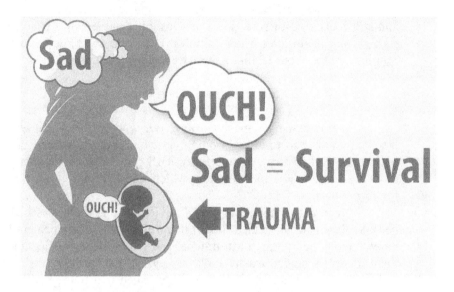

Figure 2.1: Womb trauma sets up the problem of mind chatter or 'voices' later on in life. In this example, the feeling of the mother's sadness is now linked to the feeling of survival in the fetus.

To test this idea, I found that I could get the emotional tone of a thought, regress to the same emotional tone *in my mother* while I was in the womb, and find and heal my trauma experience there. Once each prenatal trauma was healed, the corresponding 'thoughts' would vanish, leaving what felt sort of like a patch of silent emptiness in the space around me in the present.

Due to our cultural beliefs, researchers, therapists and clients for all these years had been assuming that obsessive thoughts (or mind chatter, or voices, or whatever you want to call them) must be a rejected or unconscious part of ourselves; and in the case of angry, negative thoughts, that somehow the client must be at fault due to overt or suppressed anger issues. But this approach is a complete waste of time, as far as getting rid of the voices is concerned. What I'd found showed that the content of the thoughts had *nothing* to do with the client. Instead, the thought's emotional tone was determined by the mother's feelings before the client was even born.

More background: the Hearing Voices Network

In 1987 the worldwide 'hearing voices network' (Intervoice) was founded. These were people who heard disembodied voices but had no other symptom of mental illness. My breakthrough showed that hearing voices was *not* a sign of mental illness. Instead, the only difference between these people and 'ordinary' people was that they'd simply lost the ability to mute their mind chatter. They'd simply lost their volume control. This was why researchers couldn't find a clear and obvious biological difference between the two groups – virtually everyone has the same underlying problem.

Note that the mom could have positive as well as negative feelings during the client's *in utero* trauma. For example, my mom was feeling great while having sex with dad while she was pregnant, but it left me somewhat injured. Hence, the emotional tone to that corresponding voice was very positive. As I wrote at the time:

> "Two days later, I went 'back in' to heal the other emotions that got coupled to survival – mom had positive feelings during this time, too. As I did this, I was actually able to perceive myself kicking out a cloud of 'entities' – the so-called 'angels' that surround just about everyone – into infinity. It was great, because the noise level in my head took a dramatic drop suddenly."

Dysfunctional sexual attractions and 'voices'

As you've seen in my example of being attracted to angry women, we can also eliminate these 'chunks' of mind chatter in another way. Instead of focusing on the potentially difficult task of noticing the emotional tone of thoughts that may come and go, a client could simply focus on the dominant emotional tone of each man or woman they were sexually attracted to, and use that for the regression. But why did sexual attractions matter? After all, these womb traumas had no sexual feelings – they were rather like being with your mom in a car accident. One reason has to do with how the body awareness can manipulate a person's behavior to get its way. As we've seen, the body felt its survival depended on being surrounded by the mom's emotional tones from those womb traumas. But how is it going to get its urgent survival needs met? To do this, it induces a feeling of sexual attraction towards the person who has that emotional tone. (We suspect that this sexual dynamic actually arises from conception, but as of this writing we haven't yet pursued this idea.) So, a bit like wearing a belt and suspenders, the body would want to be around any source of that emotional tone, be it an 'entity', real people, or preferably both.

Healing this in clients was fascinating. They would think about someone they were sexually attracted to, be it a movie star or someone they actually knew; notice their dominant emotional tone; regress to the corresponding womb trauma with their mom surrounding them with that same emotional tone; and heal. As soon as the trauma was eliminated, their sexual attraction for the person would just vanish and not return, along with the corresponding thought stream. It was simply amazing.

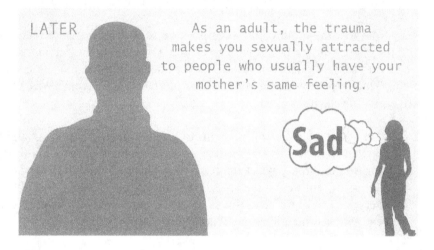

Figure 2.2: Prenatal trauma sets up dysfunctional sexual attractions as well as voices. In this example, the man is attracted to a woman who has the same flavor of sadness as his mother had when he was injured as a fetus.

Example:
A lot of interpersonal drama is caused by this problem. For example, say the *in utero* feeling of your mother was anger. So you find yourself sexually attracted to a person who also has exactly this same feeling, even though consciously you don't like being around angry people. But what happens when they start to feel something else, say happy or sad? You'll unconsciously try to make them angry again, because your body feels its survival is at stake. (Alternatively, the person might just switch to one of the other emotions you've associated with your survival. You'd still feel safe so there would be no drama.)

We've also seen children go into temper tantrums because of this – if their mom's usual emotion changes, they'll act out until the mom has her old emotion back.

Over the next decade I tested this process on many people, with exactly the same results. (People who wanted to meditate were particularly interested, as this technique would give them a permanently silent mind no matter what else they were feeling.) We would heal either the emotional tones of the thoughts in their heads, or use the emotional tones of people they were sexually attracted to. We'd continue until their minds were completely silent inside, which would usually take healing somewhere between 10 to 20 womb trauma moments.

Example:
In one interesting case the client was a sex addict. After he'd finished eliminating all his voices, his sexual cravings all vanished. It took him several months to get used to this and re-establish normal sexual relations with his wife.

Curing my Dad

My dad's schizophrenia had been getting worse and worse as the years passed. Finally, in 1987 there was no other option and he entered an extended care facility in Bonnyville, Alberta. By 1995 he was often catatonic, his teeth had all rotted out, the antipsychotic drugs had taken a terrible toll, and it was pretty clear he didn't have much longer to live. When I would visit him, I could only just to sit with him – there was no real ability to communicate anymore.

But could my new breakthrough in eliminating voices help my dad? Was this the source of his mental illness? And so he became my first test case.

The nature of his problem became almost immediately obvious. He had three very loud, evil, angry and hostile voices in his mind saying terrible things like 'kill your children'. This kind, gentle man had assumed that these voices must be his own thoughts, and had retreated from reality to escape them.

Tip for therapists:
After years of teaching therapists and physicians who work with schizophrenics, I'm continually surprised that they've never thought about what just hearing voices can do to a person. Many voice hearers are like prisoners of war being tortured with loud,

aggressive non-stop voices that continue even when they are desperate for sleep. I've often been tempted to have my students play an iPod with a high volume cacophony of spoken voices day and night for two or three days to get a small taste of what it is like. I think this might help them experientially understand a bit of the torment many voice hearers go through. For others it is the content of the voices that is the problem, like being trapped in a jail cell with a bunch of dangerous criminals who never stop threatening you - and so the client has anxiety, inability to focus attention, and so on. People with negative voices may assume that these are their own thoughts, that somehow they must be a bad person, and so try and deal with them inappropriately.

After eliminating those three voices in my dad's head – just three – he was a changed man from that day forward. As I write these words, I still have tears of happiness form in my eyes, even after all these years. You cannot imagine how it felt to get my dad back, that sane man I'd only known briefly as a child. I was now able to chat with him on the phone, ask his advice, hear his viewpoint, all things that I'd never been able to do before then. Dad became my biggest fan, even sending me money from his small annuity so I could do more research.

I later asked him what being catatonic was like, and his answer still sends chills down my back. He said it was like "being trapped in a nightmare that never ended"; I just wish I had known how to help him sooner. He died of a heart attack nine years later, just two days after receiving a copy of my first book that was dedicated to him. At his funeral, I mentioned to his sister what I'd done, and to my surprise she believed me. She'd always wondered after so many years why he'd suddenly gotten better, and what I said made sense to her.

A month before I made the breakthrough, I spoke to my brother Scott about my struggles and he said something very insightful. From my journal at the time:

> "He [Scott] said that I just had to find my own way to heal, that I couldn't depend on anyone else to do it. Scott went on to say the lesson of the Buddha was that he did it on his own, after going to all the authorities of his day. And that people now make the same mistake, going to the Buddhist authorities, etc., in a search for others just like Buddha did 2,500 years ago.
>
> "Some days, Scott impresses the hell out of me!"

Most of the people I knew during those years had tried to convince me that my intuitive feelings about the importance of trauma, and especially prenatal trauma were simply wrong. They'd espouse the virtues of their particular spiritual path, psychological technique, or simply tell me what I was hoping for was impossible. So for several years I'd stopped talking to friends and withdrew to my mountain cabin to work; I simply couldn't handle their criticisms on top of my own doubts. It wasn't easy emotionally or financially to keep going, but it somehow felt like I was on the right track, even though I had no idea where that path would finally lead.

If I'd listened to the doubts of others rather than following my own heart, I'd never have gotten my father back.

Key Points

- People should have a silent mind, one without any thoughts or chatter. This is so different from people's experience that most can't imagine living this way.
- Background thoughts (as heard during meditation) are in most cases caused by the same problem that causes the 'voices' that schizophrenics hear.
- The difference between a typical person and one who hears 'voices' is in most cases simply a matter of loss of the ability to mute the internal chatter.
- The trigger for no longer being able to suppress hearing voices is usually some traumatic event the person feels is life-threatening.
- So-called entities, angels, or channeled voices are just louder versions of normal mind chatter.

Suggested Reading

On channeling:
- *Channeling: Investigations on Receiving Information from Paranormal Sources*, Second Edition (1998), by Jon Klimo Ph.D.
- *With the Tongues of Men and Angels: A Study of Channeling* (1991), by Arthur Hastings Ph.D.

On Rogerian psychotherapy:
- *A Way of Being* (1980), by Carl R. Rogers.
- *On Becoming a Person: A Therapist's View of Psychotherapy* (1961), by Carl R. Rogers.

On trauma techniques:
- "Going for the Cure", *Family Therapy Networker* (July/August 1996), by M. D. Wylie, 20(4), pgs. 20-37. This was the first peer reviewed article about psychological techniques that could actually eliminate trauma symptoms.

On prenatal trauma:
- Association for Pre- and Perinatal Psychology and Health (APPPH), www.birthpsychology.com, www.isppm.de.
- *Primal Connections: How Our Experiences from Conception to Birth Influence Our Emotions, Behavior, and Health* (1993), by Elizabeth Noble.
- *Remembering Our Home: Healing Hurts and Receiving Gifts from Conception to Birth* (1999), by Sheila Linn, William Emerson, Denis Linn, Matthew Linn.
- *Voices from the Womb: Adults Relive their Pre-Birth Experiences – a Hypnotherapist's Compelling Account* (1992), by Michael and Marie Gabriel.

On shamanism:
- *The Way of the Shaman* (1990), by Michael Harner Ph.D.
- *Soul Retrieval: Mending the Fragmented Self Through Shamanic Practice* (1991), by Sandra Ingerman.

On the triune brain:
- *Focusing* (1982) by Dr. Eugene Gendlin. This book describes a technique for communicating with the body consciousness for psychological healing.
- *Peak States of Consciousness, Volume 1* (2004) by Dr. Grant McFetridge, Jacquelyn Aldana, and Dr. James Hardt. The triune brain model is covered from a psychological perspective.
- *The Biology of Transcendence: A Blueprint of the Human Spirit* (2002) by Joseph Chilton Pearce.
- *The Three Faces of the Mind: Developing your Mental, Emotional, and Behavioral Intelligence* (1996) by Elaine De Beauport.

Reading for professionals

Schizophrenia triggered by trauma:
- "Childhood trauma, psychosis and schizophrenia: a literature review with theoretical and clinical implications" by J. Read, J. Os, A. P.

Morrison, and C. A. Ross, *Acta Psychiatrica Scandinavica*, Volume 112:5 November 2005, pp. 330-350.
- "Delayed Post Traumatic Stress Disorder Model for Schizophrenia and Depression: The Unification Theory of Mental Illness", Dr. Clancy McKenzie M.D. 1998, *Trauma Response*, Volume 4 Number 2. Dr. McKenzie, studying thousands of schizophrenics in the USA, found that trauma in the first years of life was at the root of cause of schizophrenia in the people studied. See also "A Unification Theory of Mental Illness", 1998, *Frontier Perspectives*, Volume 7, Number 2, Temple University, Philadelphia.
- *Delayed Post Traumatic Stress Disorders from Infancy: The Two Trauma Mechanism*, by C McKenzie and LS Wright, 1996, Amsterdam: Harwood Academic Publishers.
- *Models of Madness: Psychological, Social and Biological Approaches to Schizophrenia* (2004), edited by Richard Bentall, Loren Mosher, John Read.
- "Prenatal exposure to maternal stress and subsequent schizophrenia: The May 1940 invasion of the Netherlands" by Dr.s J. van Os and J. P. Selten, (1998), *The British Journal of Psychiatry* 172:324-326. This was a key study linking prenatal trauma to schizophrenia.
- "Rates of Adult Schizophrenia Following Prenatal Exposure to the Chinese Famine of 1959-1961" (Aug 2005), by David St. Clair MD, *Journal of the American Medical Association.*
- "Trauma, Metacognition and Predisposition to Hallucinations In Non-Patients" (2003) by AP Morrison, and T Petersen, *Behavioural and Cognitive Psychotherapy*, 31: 235-246.

Voices in non-patient populations:
- "Auditory hallucinations: a comparison between patients and nonpatients" (Oct 1998) by Honig A, Romme MA, Ensink BJ, Escher SD, Pennings MH, deVries MW. *The Journal of Nervous & Mental Disease*, 186, 646–651 (Department of Psychiatry and Neuropsychology, Maastricht University, Academic Hospital Maastricht, The Netherlands).
  "The form and the content of chronic auditory hallucinations were compared in three cohorts, namely patients with schizophrenia, patients with a dissociative disorder, and nonpatient voice-hearers. The form of the hallucinatory experiences was not significantly different between the three groups."
- "Factorial Structure of the Hallucinatory Experience: Continuity of Experience in Psychotic and Normal Individuals", M Serper, CA

Dill, N Chang, T Kot, J Elliot, *Journal of Nervous and Mental Disease*, April 2005, 193(4): 265-272.

- "Psychotic symptoms in non-clinical populations and the continuum of psychosis" (March 2002), H Verdoux, Jim van Os, *Schizophrenia Research*, 54:1-2, pp 59-65.
- "The continuity of psychotic experiences in the general population", LC Johns, J van Os, 2001, *Clinical Psychology Review*, 21 (8), 1125-41

Chapter 3

The Silent Mind Technique™

The last chapter described our initial breakthrough. However, there were still many unknowns and problems with the technique. One huge difficulty was that womb traumas were intrinsically hard to face – there was always significant pain and suffering in them. Was there a better way, one where we could get rid of 'voices' all at once? More fundamentally, what was the biology behind these voices? Why could some people see 'entities' like small clouds of smoke suspended in space around themselves? Why were voices in fixed locations in space? We needed to get answers to these questions and many others before we could move forward with any kind of confidence that our techniques would be reliable and effective.

This chapter covers the key discoveries that eventually led to understanding voices at a biological level. It's also about research ups and downs, acquiring colleagues to work with in the research, and our problems with trying to introduce something entirely new into the medical community.

Discovering the primary cell

In the last half of the 1990s, my research work accelerated. I'd started participating in Kate Sorensen's groundbreaking conferences on trauma techniques and exceptional states of consciousness, where I'd had the great good fortune to be able to share data and ideas with that amazing group of altruistic technique developers. I also started to teach my Whole-Hearted Healing trauma technique to students in the US and Canada. Around 1997 or so I finally realized that I wanted to formally start my own research institute to investigate peak states, and so registered the name Institute for the Study of Peak States in British Columbia, Canada. By 1999, I was working with some truly amazing and dedicated people who became teammates in our fledging Institute: Deola Perry Ph.D., Marie Green Ph.D.,

Mary Pellicer MD, and Adam Waisel MD. With the help of students who volunteered to act as experimental subjects, each month we'd make new, important discoveries as we explored this new field of prenatal trauma and peak states of consciousness. It was an incredibly exciting time for all of us. In November of 1999, with my sister Alison's help, I made our first website (www.PeakStates.com) so we could share our discoveries and find others who shared our passion.

Meet the team - Mary Pellicer MD

Mary writes: "My lifelong commitment to healing work was inspired at the age of eight, when I witnessed the health ravages in a third world country while living there with my family. That is when I decided I wanted to help people be healthy. I trained as a family practitioner and worked for a number of years in a migrant health clinic practicing conventional medicine. I grew frustrated in that system and left to become medical director of a healthy community project for a large hospital system. Though a step in the right direction, the funding for the project was limited, compared to the need, and eventually the program was discontinued. I realized that the tools I had learned in medical school were often only band-aids for many of the chronic problems my patients had."

"In the year 1999, soon after experiencing my own peak state of consciousness, I met Grant just as he was getting the ISPS web site launched. I was intrigued, fascinated and totally hooked on researching consciousness. We worked together for 5 years until my own personal healing journey called me away. Now I am back with the Institute and excited to continue researching consciousness in the place where I started. I believe it is possible to heal anything, but in order to do so you have to be able to hack the human operating system-consciousness. Grant and the ISPS team are the best at that I know of. It's brilliant work to be involved with and a great group to be working with. Here's to healing the planet!"

The next fundamental discovery happened in the summer of 2001. During a First Nations sweat lodge ceremony on an island off the coast of British Columbia, I moved into a completely unfamiliar state of consciousness. I suddenly had acquired the ability to 'see' at will completely unfamiliar objects floating in what looked like grey mist around me. I could move my awareness around, and look up close or from a distance. I had no idea what I was seeing, but it was as visible to me as the furniture in my house.

Over the next few months, I figured out how to give my colleagues the same ability. We all started to explore this new 'spiritual' realm, and tried to figure out what it could be used for. It was about nine months later that we finally realized that we were seeing inside a cell. (Looking back, I think Adam was the first to realize this, although he says I was actually the one who figured it out. That sort of thing didn't matter to any of us; I know I felt blessed to be doing cutting-edge science with these truly gifted and dedicated colleagues.) Up to that point, none of us had a clue – electron microscope pictures of dried and sliced cell interiors were just so different from the multicolored, 3D objects we were seeing.

Over the next ten years, with the help of electron microscope photos from biology textbooks, we would slowly explore the connection between psychological symptoms, prenatal trauma and problems inside the cell. We also made one of the most surprising discoveries of our careers – there was only *one* important cell in the entire body. This cell was where consciousness itself lived, and problems in it would echo out into both other cells and into the multi-celled body structures. This cell sets the pattern and controls all other cells. We eventually called it the 'primary' cell; it forms shortly after conception.

About a third of the general population can actually 'see' reasonably well inside their own primary cell, once they are shown how. What's it like? Well, sort of like that old movie *Fantastic Voyage* (the one with Raquel Welch), where a submarine get shrunken and put inside someone's body. Once in the primary cell, just like Alice in Wonderland, you can make yourself large or small, and move wherever you want. To get a feel for what it looks like in the cell, we refer you to the YouTube video created in 2006 by Harvard University's Department of Molecular and Cellular Biology called 'Inner Life of the Cell'.

Regardless of one's ability to see inside the primary cell or not, *all* people are aware of both their physical body and their subcellular environment simultaneously – they are superimposed on each other, like some sort of video effect. *Everyone* feels problems in their primary cell in exactly the same way they feel problems in their body. This can be confusing to a person, since it isn't always obvious where the problem sensation is really coming from. (Our findings about the symptoms coming from inside the cell eventually got compiled together in the *Subcellular Psychobiology Diagnosis Handbook* in 2014.)

Being able to see structures in one's primary cell is often misdiagnosed as a visual hallucination. After all, these people are convinced that they are actually seeing something in space around themselves that no one else can see. In an era *before* electron microscopes and YouTube videos, this misdiagnosis made sense – now, it makes more sense to hire these people as walking real-time microscopes for research in subcellular biology!

The early years of the Institute

In the early 2000s the research continued, albeit schizophrenia was just a background project as we continued to focus on more fundamental questions about subcellular psychobiology. This didn't mean I was happy about this – after all, one percent of the human race is diagnosed with this disease, I certainly knew the pain this disease could cause in families and in people, and I had something that might be able to help a lot of them. But research isn't like baking a cake – breakthroughs come when they come, and to do them we had to solve more basic problems first. However, I *was* starting to train therapists in the current technique, and in 2004 Dr. Pellicer and I published *The Basic Whole-Hearted Healing Manual*. In it on pages 131-132 I described what we'd found for treating voices. (I was already planning on writing this book you have in your hands, although I had no idea it would take another 13 years!) I really wanted to get a solution out into the world, but I knew what we had wasn't good enough yet, because it really required a trained trauma therapist to use it. Nor was it yet tested on a schizophrenic population.

Two new key people had come onboard by this time: Paula Courteau (the author of the *Whole-Hearted Healing Workbook*) and John Heinegg, who had an exceptional talent for creating music for our regression work. (As I write this in 2017, I am tremendously fortunate to still be working with these two amazingly talented and dedicated people.)

Also in 2004 my first book *Peak States of Consciousness: Theory and Applications, Volume 1* was published. Suddenly, there were a lot more people interested in our work. Most were not interested in doing research – they did not understand how tough it was to develop an entirely new field of science with just a handful of volunteers on a shoe-string budget. Over the next few years I flew all over the world teaching with my colleagues. As these were the only times we could get paid to travel – we all lived in different parts of the world – trainings also became week-long intense research sessions.

2004 and 2005 were also very painful years for me. In the summer of 2004 my little sister died tragically in a car accident. That winter my dad also died, just two days after receiving a copy of my new book with its dedication to him. Then in 2005 my right-hand man, Dr. Adam Waisel died of a heart attack. Adam's death in particular was such a great blow to me that I nearly gave up the entire project. He was devoted to trying to find how to help all of humanity; a true Renaissance man, one of the smartest, most capable people I've ever met, as well as being a surgeon, an acupuncturist, and a Chinese medicine doctor. It just wasn't fun anymore without the kind of camaraderie we'd developed. But I still felt our work was important and needed doing; it just started to feel a lot more like grinding work. I also had to transition from being a colleague to being a boss as our Institute continued to grow, with all the hassles that involved. This also left less and less time for research.

Meet the team - John Heinegg

John writes: "I suppose it was meant to be. I met Grant shortly after my wife and I moved to British Columbia, in 2005. He soon discovered that I had no problem with his ideas—I was well versed in both conventional medicine (I'm a registered nurse, and make my living as a medical editor) and alternative methods (having studied a range of healing techniques sometimes derided as "woo-woo")."

"Most important, I could hear the prenatal developmental instructions as music, and had the training to reproduce that music (having been a music major in college, with a focus in composition). That mattered because of Grant's belief—soon borne out by experience—that if we had a recording of the music for a particular developmental event, and played it during a session, the client would have an easier time regressing to that event."

"I did have to learn how to create recordings of the music I heard. But thanks to computer music programs (in my case, GarageBand), nowadays a laptop attached to an electronic piano can function as a recording studio, and even a non-pianist like me can produce complex pieces."

"Early on, I sometimes found it hard to believe that I wasn't just "making it up"—was I transcribing Gaia music, or composing my own? But years of enthusiastic feedback put that to rest. I still believe that music is a language, and that someone from a non-Western musical tradition (say, classical Indian music) would hear Gaia music differently. To which the pragmatist would respond, "So what?""

"Working with Grant is a roller-coaster ride that many people can't handle for very long. Why haven't I burned out? Partly I think it's because I'm not responsible for Grant's bestiary of parasites and pathogens; I just focus on the music. And also because I've heeded that traditional warning to musicians: Keep your day job.""

Over those years I also had a steady stream of people join up and others quit. Remember, this research was extremely tough, frustrating, often physically painful, and potentially dangerous work; we were all unpaid volunteers usually with families who also (understandably enough) wanted our attention; and it usually took years to make progress on any given project as we explored this totally new and unknown biology.

Body associations and 'ribosomal voices'

As I've said, we could now 'see' inside the primary cell. But it wasn't *at all* like looking at a biology text picture with its nice little labels and arrows. It was much more like trying to identify birds flying around your house by looking at grainy black and white photos of thin slices of bird cadavers. So, if we assumed that 'voices' were actually inside the cell somewhere instead of in some intangible brain network, where should we look? Fortunately, we'd already gotten part way there. Remember those 'clouds of smoke' that some people could see when we were investigating the 'entity' phenomena? As we'd discovered, ordinary mind chatter was just muted versions of these same 'voices', so we at least had a starting point – find the 'smoke'.

We had one other important clue. Back in 2001 we'd barely started investigating the primary cell when we hit pay dirt. We found that biographical trauma was *not* caused by mental constructs in the brain, but by a *physical*, observable problem in the cell. Inside the nucleus, damaged histone proteins, acting like chewed bubblegum, were stuck to DNA genes and their messenger RNA copies, keeping these mRNA strings from going out into the cytoplasm. Technically, this is called 'inhibited gene expression'. Over the next few years, we found that the two other types of trauma - generational and associational - were also caused by this same mechanism. (A few years afterwards this same discovery of 'epigenetic damage' was being made in labs around the world; it's now one of the hottest fields in biology. But we'd also discovered something else that was even more important that, as far as we know, no one else has realized – there was a connection between trauma and epigenetics; and that epigenetic damage could be reversed by using psychological methods.)

It turned out that body associations were key to this problem of voices. To understand this, let's look at Pavlov's dog for a moment. When a bell rings, the dog salivates – that's called conditioning. Trauma can cause this conditioning via the formation of 'body associations'. That is, at the moment of trauma the body (called the reptilian brain by neurobiologists) associates a perception of its surroundings to an internal feeling - even if this makes no logical sense at all. These irrational associations can be relatively harmless, such as linking the color blue to a sensation of softness; or they can cause severe problems, as when the taste of alcohol is linked to the sensation of survival.

But what is happening biologically? The key turned out to be in the rough endoplasmic reticulum (ER), a folded membrane that surrounds most of the nucleus. When the body needs a particular protein, it would call up the right gene from the nucleus, have an mRNA copy made, then squirt the RNA string up a tube and out a pore of the ER. Once outside, a free-floating ribosome would attach to one end and pull it through itself, reading the mRNA string like a computer punch tape, and make the protein as it was reading along the string.

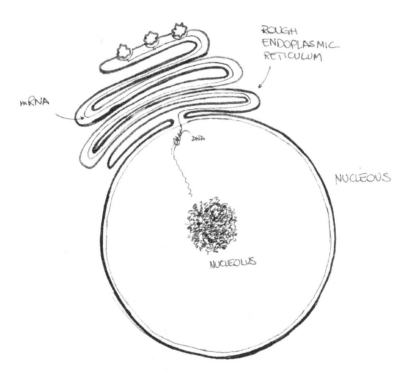

Figure 3.1: A side-view diagram of the nucleus with the rough endoplasmic reticulum (ER). An mRNA string that connects three ribosomes goes through the ER and attaches to a nuclear gene's damaged protein coating.

Well, that's if all goes well. What happens when trauma makes a body association form is quite different. In that case, the gene already has a sticky, damaged histone protein attached to it, and one end of the mRNA string gets stuck to the gene in the nucleus. The other end of the mRNA string goes up the tube and sticks out of the ER. Now, free floating ribosomes (they look a bit like empty crumpled bags) attach to the end sticking out of the ER and try to read along the mRNA, like running a computer punch tape through a reader. But they can't finish reading the information on the string as they just bang right into the ER membrane, and so settle into the ER pore, still trying to do their job. Figure 3.1 shows what this looks like in the primary cell.

But how does this involve the associational *feelings* (like hunger or salivation in the dog)? It turns out that these stuck ribosomes soak up the feelings of what was going on at that moment in time. If you put your awareness near a stuck ribosome, you find it radiates the emotion, body sensation, or both that happened in the moment of trauma (when the body needed a protein to deal with whatever was going on). Worse, every time your body wants the same protein made, a side branch on the mRNA string forms, each with a new ribosome imbedded into the ER, each with a new trauma feeling radiating from it. So over time, you can have a lot of completely random feelings and sensations tied together by this branching mRNA string in the ER.

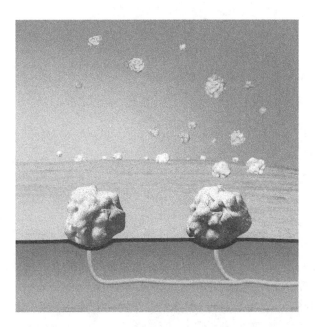

Figure 3.2: Sensations stored in these two ribosomes become associated via the connecting mRNA string in the ER membrane.

OK, now back to voices. Remember from Chapter 2 how prenatal trauma caused an *association* between rvival and the mother's emotion? It took a few years, but we finally tracked each voice to a corresponding ribosome stuck into the rough endoplasmic reticulum (ER). One could move close to the ribosome and 'hear' the voice, just like putting your ear near a cell phone, and also feel the mom's emotional tone radiating from it. And along in another ribosome connected by the mRNA string was a feeling of wanting to survive, hence the association between the two feelings. Because of this subcellular psychobiology, in our textbooks we call this type of voices '*ribosomal* voices', and they can cause anything from mild background thoughts to severe schizophrenia.

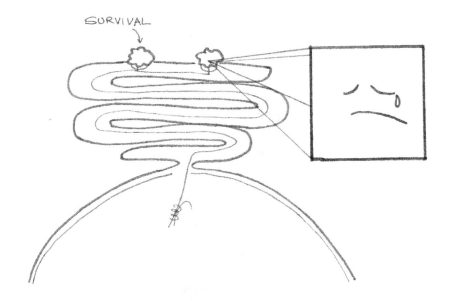

Figure 3.3: In this example, a voice is embedded in a ribosome that feels emotionally 'sad'. It connects via an mRNA string to another ribosome that contains a 'need to survive' feeling. This forms a non-logical association between the two feelings.

More background: sizes of subcellular structures

To give a feeling for just how tiny these subcellular structures are, an average ribosome has about a 20nm diameter, and an average human cell has about a 30μm diameter (with the primary cell a bit bigger at about 50μm). In terms of scale, this means we were looking for something the volume of a paperback book hidden somewhere inside the Empire State Building. Obviously, random searching just wasn't going to do the trick. (1nm = 10^{-9} meters; 1 μm = 10^{-6} meters)

Now that we'd figured out the voices were inside certain ER ribosomes in the primary cell, suddenly a lot of things made sense. We'd been healing the prenatal trauma moment to get rid of the voices, but this turned out to be overkill – all we had to do was get rid of the association, not the entire prenatal trauma. Client's 'voices' were in fixed places in space because they were imbedded in fixed places in the primary cell's ER. And the 'smoke' turned out to be how some people were sensing the interior of the ribosome that held the voice. Incidentally, some people perceive their voices outside their body, while other people hear them inside the body. This depends on how expanded the person's awareness normally is from its center inside the nucleus (the nucleus feels like the person's head). If awareness is contracted inside the nucleus, then the voices are outside their head. If their awareness is expanded past the edge of the nucleus and includes the ER, then the voices feel like they are inside the head.

We can now see why mother's emotional tone was in the ribosomes, but why were *voices* in there? And how could they be like real people you could have a conversation with? In the next chapter we'll see how we found the completely unexpected reason.

Our first global treatment – the 'Silent Mind Technique'

As you've read, our first technique for eliminating voices was both painful and difficult since it worked by healing prenatal traumas. Worse, it could only do one voice at a time. What we really wanted was a more 'global' (i.e., all at once) way to get rid of them. But this was a tough problem because we still didn't know why the voices even existed.

In June 2004 the entire international research team gathered together for the first time ever, at my home on Hornby Island. It was an extraordinary experience for all of us. During that retreat, we found a very early developmental event in the formation of the primordial germ cells (these are the cells that later become eggs or sperm) that appeared to be relevant to voices. (See Chapter 5 for details.) Assuming this was true, it meant that if a person could regress to this event and heal it, the voices should disappear. But we were sort of shooting in the dark – we'd found something that appeared connected somehow, but we had no idea why.

Over the next two years we continued revising this global technique, testing on staff then with students. To our frustration, it worked for some people but not others. We ended up calling the combination of the one-by-one and global approaches the 'Silent Mind Technique™' (SMT). But would it work with more severely ill clients? A partial answer came out of a course in Australia in 2006. One of our students had a serious problem with voices. Below is what she wrote a year after her treatment. I've included it in its entirety because it illustrates the problems and the suffering that voices can give, as well as what the outcome feels like.

"So you're wondering about the silent mind process?

"Before I had the process done I had no idea how badly I needed it. Sure I couldn't meditate if my life depended on it, and my internal life was very chaotic, but wasn't everyone like this? I talked to myself a bit (ok, a lot) (ok, all the time) and sometimes my whole day would somehow vanish in a stream of endless conversations, all in my head, but they were lucid conversations. They just never stopped. Ever.

"The inside of my mind was noisier than my 1988 university lodgings. Imagine about thirty drunk students camped out in the lounge room of your mind, yelling at each other while watching bad daytime TV, with the stereo blaring at the same time. Oh yeah, and they're all chewing pizza with their mouths open. Loudly. Imagine trying to study, work, live, love, relate and sleep in the middle of that.

"Welcome to the first thirty-six years of my life.

"Getting to sleep was torment. I've been an insomniac since I was a small child. My mind would race, churn and wind back, chattering to itself all the way. It would talk itself into countless loops. I'd eventually drift into a broken half-sleep and wake heavy, listless and unrested. It got so I'd postpone going to bed, later and later, anything to avoid lying there not sleeping, talking to myself again. I read literally thousands of books, as this was the only thing that ever shut the voices up (ok, kids, it's story time!); I read until I was so tired I'd fall asleep with the book open.

"The thing is, I didn't know any different. It's just always been like that.

"I'd tried to meditate many times, without success. 'Just let the thoughts rise, and fall away,' the meditation teacher would say. Yeah, right. My thoughts didn't fall away, ever. They'd start their own commentary on the teacher, the technique, and then they'd be off rehashing old conversations, creating new ones until it was the thought Olympics instead of Zen silence... '...guys, pay attention, I'm s'posed to be meditating...' I'd mentally hiss. There'd be order for about two seconds, then they'd start again, the unruly, undisciplined buggers. I think I managed to meditate once for about seven seconds, before the kindergarten chatter started. World record. Gold medal. Woo hoo.

"It had been like this my whole life. I thought it was normal, and I was just a bad meditator, wasn't trying hard enough, wasn't focusing. Because I didn't know any different, the voices were just background noise to the soundtrack of my life. They never told me nasty things, or were hostile or particularly mean. They were just…talkative. Helpful. Cheerful. Incessant.

"I am a bodyworker, and anyone in the healing arts will tell you that being present is an important part of the healing process. But for me being present meant hanging out with the noisy students in their non-stop party. So I developed an ability to split the awareness of my mind and body so my mind could chatter away to itself while my body got on with doing the work. I am still amazed my clients achieved any results, considering I was barely there most of the time. My body seems to really know what it's doing (after twenty years of practice, I guess it's figured a few things out) and sometimes I'd 'come to' at the end of a session and think 'oh, no, that must have been terrible, I don't even remember it' only to have the client thank me for the best session ever. Go figure.

"However there was a limit to how deep I could go with people, and I knew there was more, just had no idea how to get to it. An intensive healing search brought me to a Peak States 1 workshop in Jan 2006. On the eighth day, I achieved Silent Mind (with much-needed help from Tal… my voices weren't too thrilled with the idea of losing their identities and created havoc while I was trying to run the process. Apparently I had a stubborn version of this problem.)

"The process worked.

"I cannot even begin to convey what it was like to lie there with my mind echoing to a beautiful cathedral-like silence. For the first time in my life, I could hear the radiant emptiness of peace. I wept. 'They're gone. They're gone.' I wept some more.

"I didn't want to believe it at first in case it was a cruel trick, but no matter how hard I searched the corners of my mind, there were no voices. The students had been evicted. All that was left were a few empty pizza boxes. I walked around in wonder, listening to the silence outside, the leaves whispering against each other, so distinct, so clear. I reckoned if I listened long enough I could hear the moon.

"I haven't stopped smiling, and it was a year ago. The quality of my life has completely transformed. I am unrecognizable.

"I sat a 10-day Vipassana meditation course and meditated beautifully. My yoga practice has deepened. The healing work I've been doing has changed profoundly; not only have I incorporated some of the whole hearted healing and EFT techniques, but the level of presence I bring to each session now is solid and silent. Clients are achieving results I couldn't dream of a year ago. I am achieving results in my own healing that have never been possible before.

"I sleep. Oh, goodness, how blissful is it to say that and mean it. I sleep. My relationships have changed for the better with everyone, including my family. I am calm pretty much all the time, and the manic edge which fueled every waking minute has eased. I am much easier to be around, according to everyone I love. I am sane (well, I think I'm sane. Sane-ish?)

"I love the silence. I adore the quiet. I cherish the stillness. I won't watch tv, listen to the radio or play CD's. I don't want to break this beautiful, blessed silence. Sometimes I lie under a tree and listen outward in concentric circles, seeing how far I can hear. As I write this the only commentary I hear is the fridge, humming away. No voices.

"This change has affected every single aspect of my life in a positive way. I was in prison in a straitjacket looking through a window at freedom, with no way of touching it. Now I'm walking around in that freedom, still pinching myself that it's real. Every single day I am grateful to Grant and Tal and the whole peak states team, to everyone who has contributed to this body of knowledge, to those who have sacrificed everything to bring this level of healing to us.

"Thank you for the precious gift of silence."

(Name withheld)
February, 2007

Trying to introduce this to the health system

Every few years my colleagues or I make a bunch of calls or visits to organizations and researchers in the field of schizophrenia to try to discuss our findings with them. They are simply not interested. I still find it impossible to understand how they can act this way; in my eyes, these people should be on the lookout for any kind of new treatment at all, just in case it might actually work. After all, we were trying to give this away for *free* to help at least some of the 1% of the world's population who suffer so terribly from this disease. As I come from a field, electrical engineering, where everyone is looking for any possible way of doing a better job, I simply couldn't understand the reaction I was getting.

True, we're offering a psychological, non-drug approach to working with the voices aspect of the disease, but in my mind that was an advantage, not a drawback – no drug side effects, after all. Another huge advantage is that the changes are permanent, unlike with current drugs. There were other pluses – once people found out that this approach could work, smart people would figure out other, better ways. And trauma therapists could do it in their practice with only a minimal amount of training. What I didn't understand at the time was how radically different the paradigms of psychology and medicine are from that of engineering. Their assumption is that the only possible solution for serious mental disorders must be drugs, as psycho-immunological techniques are just a fantasy (or at best only involve minor stress relief).

More background: schizophrenia drug treatments

If you are a layperson reading this book and don't know anything about schizophrenia, you might assume that the pharmaceutical industry has developed reliable treatments for schizophrenia, so these patients just need to "take their meds". Sadly, that is not the case. Psychiatrists divide the symptoms of schizophrenia into four categories: positive (such as voices), negative (such as inertia), cognitive, and mood. Antipsychotic drugs only affect the positive symptoms, and they often cause serious side effects. And they simply may not work. Many research studies of antipsychotic therapy for schizophrenia track the number of patients who stop taking the drug because it isn't effective or it causes intolerable side effects—and that number is substantial. Even if they do stay on the drug, as many as 20% of people with schizophrenia may suffer relapses. The closing of mental hospitals during the 1970s was a way of saving money, not because there was a solution to the disease. The book *Surviving Schizophrenia*, by Dr. E. Fuller Torrey is an excellent source for both current and historical viewpoints and specifics on this disease.

I'll give an example of this problem. In 2007, I went into town and met the manager of our local health office that worked with schizophrenics. John Heinegg and I proposed that we treat two volunteers who had schizophrenia with our non-invasive, psychological approach. We would have one of their staff supervise and test for any improvements. If it worked, we would write to the central office to ask them if they would be interested in following up this with a more rigorous study. She thought this sounded reasonable, and so we proceeded with the test. It worked moderately well – this early process only got rid of voices but didn't fix other mental health issues – so we wrote up our proposal with her endorsement. I was stunned by their reply: the psychologist in charge of pilot studies refused to even consider our proposal, because he said that any non-drug approach was clearly unethical since schizophrenics required continuous treatment with drugs.

In a similar vein, in 2007 the Schizophrenia Society of Canada also rejected our proposal and said this about our approach: "SSC believes that schizophrenia is indeed a mental illness that involves genetics and environmental factors. Furthermore the position of SSC is that schizophrenia is treated through various treatment options of which medication is "the chief cornerstone."

As of this writing (2017), no health organization or academic institution in North America has been willing to even consider the approach we've taken. Amazingly enough, this rejection also includes faculty members who have successfully used our technique on themselves. By contrast, we've had at least some interest in the EU, although nothing has come of it yet.

The Scottish Schizophrenia Clinic

In the spring of 2008, some of my students decided to move forward with schizophrenia. These five, very enthusiastic volunteers (who had a whole range of professional backgrounds) wanted to apply the techniques I'd developed and open a clinic to help schizophrenia-diagnosed patients in Scotland. I flew from Canada and spent three months teaching and working on the project with them.

Although we were able to help some of our clients, the results were generally disappointing to all of us. We only had one clear win out of more than ten clients, although several others had improvements. The technique that had worked so well on my dad only worked marginally on these clients, if at all. This was a very painful example of the problem of doing research and development in a new field – projections and schedules can run afoul of factors that are completely outside one's control. I'd had good success in small-scale testing, but when we moved to a larger group of very sick individuals, our projected success rate did not pan out.

I spent much of those months trying to improve my understanding of the disease. The problem was that we were using only a ribosomal ER and prenatal trauma model for the voices. We didn't really have any idea of their underlying cause; all we really had was just one slow, difficult method to get rid of them. But towards the end of our time there, I got very, very lucky. During a session, our test case suddenly got an entirely new voice - and watched how it happened. She witnessed in her primary cell an octopus-like thing stick a tentacle into a ribosome, and suddenly she could hear a new voice. This was a eureka moment for me, as I'd seen that organism before; and although it didn't save the clinic, this observation would eventually help unlock the problem, as we'll see in the next chapter.

Sadly, we all went our separate ways soon after, as we all felt pretty disheartened by our failure.

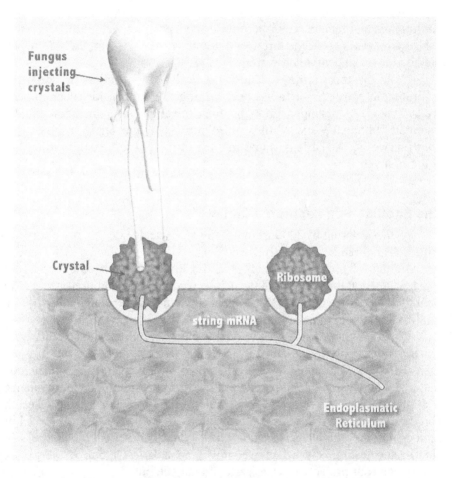

Figure 3.4: A borg fungus injecting crystals into a ribosome in the endoplasmic reticulum (not to scale). This is the origin of a 'voice'.

Meditation and the 'Listening to Silence' state

In the previous chapter, I mentioned how this work with schizophrenia was really triggered by the idea that making one's mind silent in some way other than with meditation might be a way to get profound peak states. This and an investigation into channeling eventually led to the silent mind technique I just spoke about.

But it turns out that I'd missed a completely different phenomenon involving meditation. (In hindsight, that was probably a good thing, otherwise I'd never have investigated schizophrenic voices.) Our work was a lot like voyaging centuries ago to map unknown corners of the world. Thus, to move my projects forward, I kept exploring: meditating, finding new prenatal developmental events, sharing with peers in the field, and just about anything else I could think of. And occasionally this triggers something new, either at the time or a bit later. This was an example of the 'bit later' case. I was walking outside my home one day around 2004 when I was suddenly filled with the deepest inner peace and silence I'd ever felt. This lasted for days, then gradually faded away. I felt like I was focused inward, somehow 'listening' to the deepest, most profound silence possible. Because of this, I called it the 'Listening to Silence' state.

This could explain a lot about meditation practices. This state of consciousness shuts off every type of inner noise in a person, *but* if they stop meditating, the state is lost and the mind chatter starts up again. A bit like a lot of drugs – you quit taking them, the symptoms return. As a technique for healing schizophrenia, it would only be a temporary fix unless one could make the state be permanent.

Well, this got my attention, but it wasn't until 2009 or so that I was able to duplicate it in my staff and understand what caused the state. To explain the next bit, I'm going to explain a key discovery that Dr. Pellicer made in 2005. She noticed that if you asked people to point to where in their body they feel they are, different people point to different areas, or even to more than one area. (We actually have them take their finger, point above their head, and then slowly move their finger downwards until it is pointing at 'them'.) This was incredibly exciting, as it allowed us to define consciousness with a kinesthetic process! We ended up calling this the 'center of awareness' (CoA). (We later discovered that the CoA was a physical substance located inside the primary cell; conscious awareness is a property of this material.)

If a person was able to move their CoA into their solar plexus *and* hook into what feels like an anchoring point there, they would get the state. Some people had a tougher time, the most common reason being their CoA was split into left and right pieces and they'd have to get both of themselves into the anchor spots, but the principle was the same. The real problem –

none of my test subjects could make it stable. Soon their CoA would move away from the solar plexus and they'd loose the state. This instability also explained why meditators need to keep meditating to retain their state. (It wasn't until 2017 that we started to realize why the state was unstable, and it involves two very early, very complex developmental events, ones outside the scope of this book.) Worse, without the concept of a kinesthetically identifiable CoA, meditation teachers cannot explain to their students exactly what they should do to get this state, making even momentary success very hit or miss.

I've included this fascinating discovery because I think that you, like myself, needed to understand how the meditative approach and the 'voices' approach are independent of each other. Sometimes meditation can temporarily give a person a 'quiet mind' – but as we'll be seeing in a later chapter, this only bypasses a major underlying fungal disease problem.

Key Points

- A single 'primary' cell sets the pattern for all cells in the body. A person's consciousness resides in this cell.
- People's symptoms are an overlay of sensations from their body (our normal experience) with feelings from *inside* the primary cell.
- Illogical associations between various sensations and emotions are caused by ribosomes imbedded in the endoplasmic reticulum (ER) membrane.
- Background thoughts and 'voices' are found inside ribosomes imbedded in the ER. We call them 'ribosomal voices'.
- The 'Silent Mind Technique' is a collection of processes to eliminate ribosomal voices and other related problems.
- Most health systems have an institutional bias toward ongoing drug treatment and against psychological techniques for schizophrenia.
- The 'center of awareness' (CoA) concept uses body sensations to experientially define consciousness by finding its physical location in a person.
- The 'Listening to Silence' state of consciousness is characterized by profound silence inside a person. It occurs when their CoA is anchored into their solar plexus.

Suggested Reading

About schizophrenia:

- *Surviving Schizophrenia: A Family Manual*, 6th edition (2013) By E. Fuller Torrey M.D. The best book we know of on the topic. A must read for suffers and the family of sufferers.
- "Case Study: Eliminating Schizophrenic 'Voices' by Healing Prenatal Trauma" (Aug. 2007), by Grant McFetridge Ph.D, *Positive Health (PH) Magazine*, Issue 138.
- *Psychological Disorders: Schizophrenia* (2007) by Heather Barnett Veague, Ph.D.

About the primary cell:

- *Peak States of Consciousness*, Vol. 2 (2008) by Grant McFetridge Ph.D. and Wes Geitz.
- *Subcellular Psychobiology Diagnosis Handbook* (2014) by Grant McFetridge Ph.D.

About the 'center of awareness' (CoA):

- *The Basic Whole-Healing Healing Manual* (2004) by Grant McFetridge Ph.D. and Mary Pellicer MD. This book briefly describes the CoA technique, and the prenatal traumas that create voices.
- *Peak States of Consciousness*, Vol. 2 (2008) by Grant McFetridge Ph.D. and Wes Gietz. See chapter 5 for a more in-depth discussion of the CoA phenomena.

About generational epigenetic damage:

- *The Ghost in your Genes* (Video, 2005) by the British Broadcasting Corporation. This film does an excellent job of explaining Dr. Pembrey's discovery of generational epigenetic damage via data from families in an isolated town in Sweden.
- "Transgenerational epigenetic inheritance: how important is it?" (March 2013), *Nature Review Genetics*, 14, 228-235, by Ueli Grossniklaus, William G. Kelly, Anne C. Ferguson-Smith, Marcus Pembrey, and Susan Lindquist.

Chapter 4

The Fungal Origin of Ribosomal Voices

In the last chapter we finally saw the 'smoking gun' – a new voice had appeared in a client when a fungus inside the cytoplasm stuck a filament into an ER ribosome. In this chapter, we'll look more closely at this fungus and how it indirectly makes voices. We'll see how the voices appear, and where they go when the right prenatal trauma is healed. We'll also see why you can have a conversation with these disembodied ribosomal voices as if you were talking to an actual person.

We'll also look at some of the strange, usually discounted observations made over the years about schizophrenia that now suddenly make sense: voices heard by people who are deaf from birth; voices speaking in foreign languages; and isolated populations without schizophrenia until contact with the West.

The implications of this pandemic fungal disease in the mentally-well population are even more profound. Most disturbingly, this subcellular fungal parasite has the ability to manipulate the mental state and behavior of its host. It affects day-to-day behaviors, particularly in the areas of relationships and some physical diseases or symptoms.

This widespread fungal disease has also been the direct cause of societal problems in our species. It is the source of racism, cross-cultural conflicts, wars, and dysfunctional cultural norms and behaviors. Eliminating this organism, perhaps by finding a drug or a vaccine to immunize people against it would dramatically change our world.

Resistance to acquiring peak states

I'm going to back up a bit, to talk about another investigation we were doing that at the time seemed to be completely unrelated to voices.

After the publication of my first book about peak states of consciousness in 2004, I started teaching what we'd discovered so far. My team and I had come up with some experimental techniques that could actually give people different peak states, and so we started to test these with student volunteers. Many of these enthusiastic men and women would use our technique and get the wonderful new feeling of the target peak state. But then we immediately started to see something that completely baffled us. Right after treatment, their enthusiasm would shut off like a light switch and they would just quit. They no longer had any interest in getting a second wonderful peak state from our list. This made absolutely no rational sense, as at this point, they knew from their own experience that these processes worked. We came up with a lot of ideas to try to explain this behavior, but nothing really fit.

It was in the fall of 2004 in Portland, Oregon when I got a first glimpse of the answer. While standing on the sidewalk chatting with one of these suddenly apathetic students, I noticed something. Just thinking about getting a new peak state caused us both to feel like there was suddenly a burden pushing down on us, like wearing a heavy backpack. In my case, it had been there for years and I'd just ignored it. But in my student, it was shutting down his natural enthusiasm. Fortunately, I was able to immediately track down the cause. We both had the sensation of negative, painful emotions coming into our navels from outside our body when we thought about getting new peak states. In the student's case, as soon as he stopped thinking about wanting a peak state, the painful feelings and heaviness would also stop. The tradeoff was that his innate goals and enthusiasm were also lost.

The 'Tribal Block'

Over time, we found this strange mechanism in almost everyone we checked. Worse, it wasn't just about having peak states – it permeated people's entire lives. Disturbingly, it actually dominates their decision-making process in all kinds of areas. For example, if a person wanted to do something that their family, community, or country didn't want them to do, they would be hit with painful emotions to get them to go back into their socially approved role. (When one 'looked' out the navel, one commonly saw or felt 'people' they knew, or a sense of many people, all sending a strong emotion at the client. Some might see objects, colors or patterns instead.) The feelings coming into one's navel could be virtually anything, from nasty to nice. It was like watching someone being conditioned – pain to avoid something, pleasure to do something else. We soon realized that most people had learned to automatically obey early in their lives. These people were like well-trained horses; a small flick of the reins keeps the horse on the trail, away from the lush grass nearby. We ended up calling this phenomenon the 'tribal block'. 'Tribal' because it involved issues from a person's tribe, ranging from their immediate family to social groups to their entire nation; and 'block' because it blocked people's true positive nature with social conditioning. In 2005 we developed the 'Tribal Block Technique™' that allowed us to eliminate this influence on a per-issue basis (see Appendix E for the steps). In extensive testing over the last 17 years, we've found that almost everyone has the tribal block problem, irrespective of country of origin or ethnicity. This is a species-wide problem; it is not restricted to just a few therapy clients.

> *Example – high-functioning people*
> This problem is especially noticeable in high-functioning people, those who are generally productive, calm and happy with their lives. When people like this come in for therapy, it is usually because of only one problem - they want to do something, usually altruistic, that the tribal block is opposed to. This makes them feel weighed down, struggling, and confused. Fortunately, this is easy to eliminate using the Tribal Block Technique.

But why does this problem exist at all?

Back then, we were still getting used to the idea of looking inside the primary cell for biological causes to psychological problems. And sure enough, the cause of the tribal block was in the cell. We eventually tracked it to a species of fungus that looks a lot like an octopus. In just about everyone there are a lot of them floating in the cytoplasm and attached to the outside of the cell membrane. Biologically, it sends feelings into a person by inserting a filament into a biographical trauma ribosome to stimulate the feeling stored in it (see the figure below). It's a bit like pulling a rope to ring a bell. Because of its ability to control people's actions, we started calling it the 'borg' fungus (as in the science fiction show Star Trek with its 'borg collective' that tries to assimilate and control entire species).

Because this fungal parasite's influence is so pervasive (yet unrecognized) in everyday life, one can pick virtually any topic a person wants to think about and use the Tribal Block Technique on it. This quickly demonstrates to people both the existence of this parasite infection and its powerful controlling influence on their lives. And this has the added bonus that interested readers can easily find out for themselves if what we've said is really true or not.

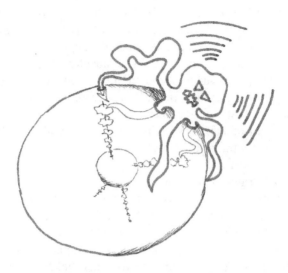

Figure 4.1: The borg fungus stimulating trauma inside the primary cell. In this example, one organism is shown attached to the outside of the cell (not to scale) with tentacles penetrating the cell membrane and extending almost to the nucleus. (There are also many borg living fully inside the cell.)

More background: host manipulation by parasites
When we first discovered that a fungal parasite could influence and even control human emotions and behavior, we were shocked. Worse, we believed that this finding would never be accepted, and our work discounted or ignored. But the world changes. In the years since our discovery, the fact that parasites can control other species behavior has become accepted in the field of parasitology and known by the public. Films of ants being controlled by fungus, bacteria making mice attracted to cats, the list goes on and on.

In humans, the fact that gut bacterial or the candida fungus can influence our eating choices is now accepted. Realizing there are probably other diseases that can psychoactively affect people is a small jump; albeit recognizing *subcellular* diseases could potentially cause this problem is still a big hurdle.

Cultural norms and cross-cultural conflicts

And then we found this 'borg' fungus causes an even worse problem.

These parasitical organisms are aware, and have an agenda that was *not* about helping their host. As we experimented, we came to realize these fungal organisms share a single 'group mind' awareness. They are more like cells in a distributed 'body' than individual creatures. Their body is made up of the fungal cells in *all* people infected with that particular pathogen. And their awareness is completely non-human; they view people as simple living space, a bit like you might view a bunch of cheap RVs. From a human perspective, this fungus is like a psychopath, with complete disregard for the suffering or death of its hosts.

Remember the perception of the emotions coming into the navel from outside? This happens because one of the fungal cells is attached in the subcellular equivalent of the navel, acting a bit like a placenta. And this one gives a person the unconscious assumptions of one's culture. We soon realized, since we had an international research team, that people from different cultures were infected by different borg fungal sub-species. The fungus from people in one culture all share the same awareness, while people from another culture are infected with a fungus that has a different awareness. And multicultural people carry two (or more) borg sub-species in their primary cell that they would switch between (or try to reject) when they were in the different cultures. To our shock, we'd discovered that cultural identity and cross-cultural antagonism is an artifact of the borg infection. Our history, filled with its bloody national and racial wars and conflicts, are the direct result of attempts by this fungus to expand its territory (in more humans) at the expense of others in its species.

Example – multicultural clients
We've seen clients who reject their birth culture, who find any attempts to visit again repulsive and difficult. These people can often sense their birth culture radiating from somewhere on or in their body. Eliminating their fungal infection immediately solves this issue, with the client no longer having a problem with their birth culture.

More background: stages of cultural adjustment
This fungal infection explains why people who attempt to join another culture ('cultural adjustment') can feel panic that they are at risk of dying and need to run away. If the person perseveres, in a moment their anxiety will suddenly end and they will suddenly 'know' the unconscious rules of their new culture. From a biological view, this is the moment they become infected with a different borg sub-species.

A significant percentage of the population (perhaps 20-30%) go even further. They consciously or unconsciously surrender or merge their awareness with the fungal parasite. This makes them feel powerful (because they feel powerless in themselves) or safe or both. These people tend to be rigid in their thinking (extremists of any stripe), and live out the fungal parasite perspective, viewing others without normal human compassion.

In 2011 we finally came up with a reliable way, using regression and generational trauma healing techniques, to make people immune to the borg fungus (see Chapter 5). One of the most fascinating results to me showed up while travelling through international airports. Up to that point, there was always a sense of people from other cultures being different and in some cases unpleasant. After the treatment, suddenly *everyone* was the same, they just wore different clothes, hair or had different body appearances. The overlay of the fungal antagonism to others of its species was gone.

At this point, you the reader might be shaking your head about all this. It certainly sounds delusional! But remember, we had a decade to get used to this as we slowly worked it out – you've gotten it cold in just a few pages. But happily the techniques work, the kinesthetic symptoms are easily felt, and so this material is useful regardless whether you accept our subcellular biology explanation or not.

Transference, 'cords' and 'curses'

It turns out that the borg fungus causes yet another species-wide problem.

While living in California in the 1980s, I heard a lot of talk about 'cords' in the alternative healing community. The idea was that somehow people were unconsciously interacting at a distance and causing each other problems. Sort of like transference and counter-transference, but not through speech or body postures. I would just roll my eyes, since it was all obviously nonsense. Even more embarrassing, a few were even foolish enough to talk about 'curses' as if they were real, something right out of cheap Hollywood movies.

But I was wrong - these phenomena do actually exist, albeit not for the reasons these people believed. This problem shows up in the dysfunctional ways people interact in professional and personal relationships. So, what does this problem feel like? If a person thinks about another, they usually identify them by an emotional sense of their 'personality', generally a negative or positive one. Remember my story about being attracted to angry women in Chapter 2? Those women not only acted angry, but to me they 'felt' angry when I put my attention on them.

Normally we consider another's 'personality' to be some sort of construct in our mind that we've made about the other person, but this turns out to be incorrect. Instead, it is a *real-time* experience of the other person at a distance. How do we know? Shortly we'll describe the technique that demonstrates this, but to understand it we first need to review the fascinating underlying subcellular biology of biographical trauma (i.e., traumatic memories from physically or emotionally painful moments in our lives).

When something happens in our lives, the cells respond by making particular proteins to do the job. To make a protein, a DNA gene is 'expressed'; it is unwound from the nucleolus (a bundle of DNA strands that looks a bit like a ball of yarn), and brought to the inner surface of the nucleus. There, a histone protein coating on the gene is stripped off (like removing the plastic insulation from a copper wire), and an mRNA copy is made. The mRNA goes out a nuclear pore and into the cytoplasm (like throwing string out a porthole of a ship). A ribosome then attaches to one end and starts reading the mRNA like an old-style computer punch tape. As it reads the string, step-by-step it makes the desired protein. That is what happens when all goes well.

As with body associations described in a previous chapter, the problem occurs because the coating on the gene is defective. An mRNA copy is made but gets stuck to this coating. But unlike body associations, the other end of this mRNA string goes directly out the nuclear pore, a ribosome finds it, and starts running down the string. But now the ribosome bangs into the nuclear membrane – it can't complete its job of making a protein. Worse, this setup freezes in place. But how does all this relate to trauma? Isn't it stored in the brain? No, the stuck ribosome acts like a *gateway* through time to that past traumatic moment, with the emotional content stored in the gene's stuck histone.

So, rather than outer circumstances creating biographical trauma (as seems reasonable), outer circumstances just trigger the need for a histone-damaged gene that then creates a stuck mRNA string with a ribosome containing the trauma moment. The next time circumstances require the same protein, yet another ribosome attaches to the string, runs down it, bangs into the first ribosome, and now another trauma moment is created (see figure 4.2). This explains why some people are unaffected by an event that can devastate others – one has a gene with a normal histone coating, while the other person's gene histone was defective (inherited or damaged during conception). Over a lifetime, we see a lot of ribosomes on a stuck mRNA string, each corresponding to a traumatic memory, all containing the same emotional tone. These strings accumulate on the outer surface of the nucleus, and from a distance look a lot like a seaweed forest on an ocean floor.

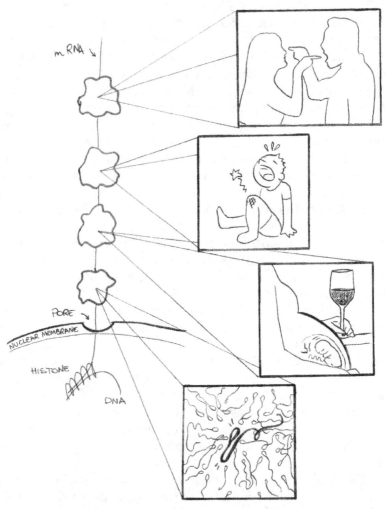

Figure 4.2: A stuck ribosome string with a biographical traumatic memory embedded inside each ribosome. The mRNA string is stuck to a gene inside the nucleus.

Now, back to 'cords'. When we interact with another person, be it someone we know or a total stranger, we may also unconsciously interact through the borg fungus. Remember, each of these fungal organisms is interconnected as one super-organism. What we see when a cord forms is that a borg fungal tentacle (or as a biologist would call it, a fungal hypha) attaches to a biographical trauma ribosome. The name 'cord' comes from a perception of this hollow tentacle. The feeling in that trauma is passed via the parasite to another parasite in the second person's primary cell. That parasite in turn has a tentacle stuck into a biographical trauma ribosome. In essence, the trauma ribosomes act like cell phones with the fungus acting like the cell towers. And these are not just random traumas – the connection is between complementary traumas. For example, an abuse trauma is tied to an abuser's trauma, a disapproval trauma is attached to a disapproving trauma, and so on.

We didn't understand this biology at first. Instead, around 1998 or so I came up with a technique that actually changed what the other person's personality felt like. We called this the 'Distant Personality Release™' technique. It was only years later that we were able to watch what it was doing inside the primary cell. The technique dissolves the mRNA 'trauma' string with its collection of ribosomes in the other person as well as in the person doing the process. If the technique is used to completion, the entire stuck gene assembly in both people is released. To the person using the technique, it feels like the other person's personality changes. In cases where there are a lot of these fungal interconnections, it may take a number of repeated uses to dissolve all of the trauma strings interconnections, each with its own personality feeling. In the end, it is like the other person no longer has any personality and vanishes from your perception. (Incidentally, this phenomenon is not a projection; those are caused by a totally different biological mechanism.)

More background: unconditional love

While I was living in Hawaii in 1997, I decided to investigate unconditional love, which was a popular topic during those years in the new age community. I focused on feeling it for a while, but no special insights arose. A few days later I was outside eating a fish taco when a car with several young guys drove up. They were all smoking, something I detest because my folks smoked when I was young. However, this time I suddenly felt a wave of love for them, which as you might imagine greatly surprised me! I put this experience in the back of my mind and continued on with other projects.

A year or two later I was focusing on my current girlfriend whose personality felt quite negative and judgmental to me. The memory of those smokers came to mind, and I suddenly saw a way to use that feeling of unconditional love to help her. Trying it, her personality quickly changed in my perception; but was replaced by another feeling that I didn't like either. I laugh now looking back, but it took another month before I was willing to unconditionally love this new feeling I felt in her; and again her personality changed.

Over time I was able to turn my intuitive actions into steps that most people could also do fairly easily – this became the Distant Personality Release (DPR) technique. *The Basic Whole-Hearted Healing Manual* (2004) goes into this process in great detail (pages 75-86) with the steps and risks that we've seen with using this technique.

In summary, a therapist can eliminate a cord on a one by one basis, or all at once (along with all potential future cords) by making a person immune to the borg fungus.

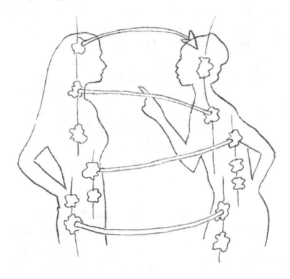

Figure 4.3a: Experiential 'cord' connections between two people's ribosomal trauma strings.

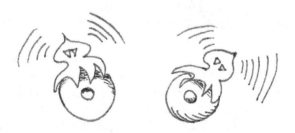

Figure 4.3b: Biologically, the 'cords' are the tentacles of borg fungi in each person's primary cell. Borg fungi in different people act a bit like cell phones, making a borg-to-borg communication link. This gives the sensation of a continuous cord stretching between two physically separated people.

But what about 'curses'? It turns out that a trauma in one person can drive the borg fungus in the other person's cytoplasm to form something that looks like a black, obsidian 'shard' (attached to a fungal tentacle). This shard can cause physical pain, but its biggest effect is from its content – it influences a person's body to act in ways that can affect emotional or physical health. This problem is far less common in the general population, and for the most part dissolve quickly when the two people stop interacting. The treatment is the same as for cords.

Now we're finally ready to get back to ribosomal voices...

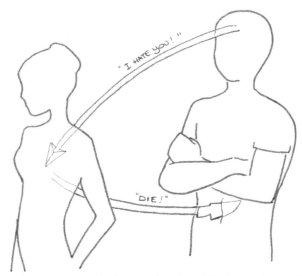

Figure 4.4a: An experiential sketch of a shard-looking object (the 'curse') attached to 'cords' sent from another person. The borg fungi in different people act as the interconnection mechanism, giving the illusion of a continuous cord connection through space between people.

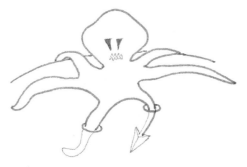

Figure 4.4b: Biologically, the curse is a shard-like structure in the cytoplasm attached to a borg fungal tentacle. In this example, the borg

fungus is shown on the outside of the cell membrane, with the curse on the lower right tentacle inside the cell membrane.

The fungal origin of ribosomal voices

In the last chapter, we saw that a new ribosomal voice was made in a client when a filament from a free-floating organism inserted itself into an ER ribosome. And as you may have guessed, we immediately recognized the organism as a borg fungus, the same one that causes the tribal block phenomenon. So what we thought of as two completely unrelated problems were actually caused by the same disease. We were eventually able to prove this when we developed a reliable technique to make people immune to this disease. The treatment silenced the mind, *and* it also got rid of the tribal block and cultural hyper-awareness problems.

Over the next year or two we looked more closely at how this fungus was actually creating the ribosomal voices. What we saw was very strange. The fungus was injecting a piece or perhaps small pieces of what looked like translucent white crystal into the ribosome (see figure 3.4). These crystal bits contain the voice. Thus, when our techniques dissolve a ribosome that contains a voice, the ribosome is released into the cytoplasm and dissolved, or parts of it are dissolved *in situ* in the ER pore. The crystals inside are now disposed of, by ejection from the cell or returned to the fungus, we don't know which.

Does this parasite crystalline material make a radio-like connection to a living person who at some unconscious level becomes the voice? Or does this crystalline material contain some kind of person-analog with all their memories and ability intact? From an engineering viewpoint, I strongly suspect the former. Since these borg parasites interconnect to a *lot* of people, it makes the radio-like hypothesis much more likely, but we simply don't know. Regardless, we have techniques that work, making this question academic albeit fascinating. (As my colleagues used to say, questions like this are why God invented graduate students...)

More background: fungal 'group minds'

Incidentally, we've found that there are a lot of completely different fungal parasite species in the primary cell, each causing very different kinds of problems. What characterizes all of them is the presence of various types of crystalline material inside their fungal bodies. For the most part, these bits of crystal act sort of like radios. In the case of the borg fungus, we believe that it uses crystalline material to be connected as a single awareness with multiple bodies.

It is clear that the fungal bodies in different people don't communicate to each other chemically, because it happens instantaneously over many miles. And it is unlikely that it happens via EM radiation, as the fungal structures are far too tiny. Some kind of quantum entanglement via the crystalline material is the most likely mechanism.

This also explains the rather unbelievable finding that people who were deaf from birth can sometimes still 'hear' audible voices. People are not hearing the voices with their ears. Instead, they are 'hearing' the voices in the crystalline bits via connection through their own ER and ribosomes. People's awareness is in the primary cell, and we sense whatever is inside it.

The existence of ribosomal voices also explains how some people report that they hear some of their voices speaking in a foreign language, often one that the person doesn't even know. If you assume that the voice is an artifact of the person's brain, then this doesn't make any sense and must therefore be a mistake or some kind of deception. However, if you recognize that the voices have absolutely no connection to the person hearing them, but instead are a kind of connection to other people, this suddenly makes sense; and in fact could even be predicted to exist.

The other epidemiological finding that supports our statement that ribosomal voices are caused by a fungal disease is something that many in the field don't know. Voices as we see them today are often completely unknown in isolated populations that have had no contact with Europeans. As Dr. Torrey in his book *Surviving Schizophrenia* points out, around the 1950s this sort of data started to simply be ignored in the textbooks, as it didn't support the belief at the time that voices were due to some kind of problem in the brain, and not due to a communicable disease. (In my own training, my abnormal psychology textbook pointed this fact out, but I didn't hear any further mention of it for the rest of my career.)

Even more interesting is that the percentage of people with mental illness and voices as we see them today has been rising in the last century. But as Dr. Torrey's points out, this problem didn't really show up in Europe until the late 1700s. So, if ribosomal voices are from a widespread fungal disease that very likely has been infecting humans for thousands of years (as we will see in the next chapter), then why this change? I can think of several possibilities. Perhaps the organism has mutated over time, or a more virulent strain was encountered somewhere in the world by sailors in the 1700s and spread. It is also possible that there is another contributing problem – the way birth is now handled. In our work with peak states, we've found that roughly 4/5 of the children whose umbilical cord is cut long after birth are *significantly* more mentally healthy than children whose cords are cut immediately at birth. Among other problems, this 'cord cutting trauma' blocks feelings of wholeness and increases feelings of loneliness and suicide in most people. Since we've seen that loneliness can trigger the acquisition of new voices, it is not too far fetched to suspect this is having an impact on the current statistics. Of course, the rise in serious mental illness may be due primarily to other disease processes, some of which we'll cover in Chapter 7.

More background: characteristics of people who 'hear voices'
The International Hearing Voices Network (Intervoice) founded by Romme, Escher and Hage does an excellent job of identifying research that shows many people hear voices but are not mentally ill. Romme and Escher (2001) write "only 16% of the whole group of voice hearers can be diagnosed with schizophrenia". They call out the following points that our discovery of ribosomal voices explains:

- Studies have found that between four and 10 per cent of people across the world hear voices.
- Between 70 and 90 cent of people who hear voices do so following traumatic events.
- Voices can be male, female, without gender, child, adult, human or non-human.
- People may hear one voice or many. Some people report hearing hundreds, although in almost all reported cases, one dominates above the others.
- Voices can be experienced in the head, in the ears, outside the head, in some other part of the body, or in the environment.

Meet the team - Nemi Nath

Nemi writes: "I joined the team in 2005 or 2006. Grant found an article of mine on the internet that resulted in me reading his book. I am not a great reader, only read what really interests me. My response to the book was: here is someone putting into words many things I had observed in my 25 years of Breathwork practice and I got a sense of direction where to go with my own findings. I only move on in life when I know it to be my path." [*Editor's note:* Ms. Nath is a past president of the International Breathwork Foundation, and ran her international school for breathwork from 1985-2008 in NSW Australia.]

Meet the team – Nemi Nath
(continued from previous page)

"The change from Breathwork to PeakStates work was bumpy at times as change often is. Sometimes I felt that I had never done any healing on myself when encountering early developmental events... being part of the research team, digging into unexplored, new biological territory can be relentless... and there is only one way for me, forward. Letting go of outmoded healing concepts and developing whatever works and helps changing humanity toward the Good.

"I love working with clients, trying to figure out why something is not working and finding solutions, and I love developing trainings and getting the work out to the people and into mainstream. We are not meant to suffer as humans because we have the potential to embody mental health and ordinary and extraordinary positive states of consciousness. That is what I am here to support. My motto is: I am committed to doing this until it is no longer needed on the planet... then I will listen to what is next."

Key Points

- A subcellular fungus in the primary cell indirectly causes ribosomal voices in people.
- This fungus also influences behavior in people by evoking positive and negative emotions. People change their thoughts and behavior to make the feelings stop. Because of this, we nicknamed this species the 'borg' fungus.
- This fungus directly causes global social issues like war, racism, and cultural hypersensitivity.
- Several different types of problems in typical therapy clients are due to various aspects of this fungus.
- Ribosomal voices arise from crystals injected into ER ribosomes by this fungus.
- Most people experience organisms and objects in their primary cell as if they were part of themselves. These organisms can cause audible, visible, and kinesthetic experiences.

- Realizing that a fungal disease causes ribosomal voices explains phenomena about voices no one has understood: voices heard by deaf-from-birth people; voices that speak in other languages that the person does not know; and isolated tribes that don't have voices until contact with the larger infected cultures.
- The Hearing Voices Network is a worldwide organization working to explain that voices are not usually a sign of mental illness, but instead something that is much more common in the general public than has been assumed.

Suggested Reading

Deaf people hearing voices:
- "Hallucinations in Deaf People with a Mental Illness: Lessons from the Deaf Clients" (1999), by D Briffa, *Australasian Psychiatry*, 7(2) pp 72-74. Some people deaf from birth report hearing 'voices'.
- "Hearing about the voices of the deaf" (2005), in Psychminded.co.uk. A popularized article about people with this condition.

Voices not present in isolated populations:
- *The Institutional Care of the Insane of the United States and Canada* (1916), pg. 381. In 1827-9 there was no evidence of any mentally ill Cherokee before or during the period of their forced relocation (the trail of tears).
- *Surviving Schizophrenia: A Family Manual*, 6th edition (2013) by E. Fuller Torrey M.D. See Chapter 1 for a discussion on the appearance of voices only in the last few centuries.

Stages of 'cultural adjustment':
- *Returning Home* (1984), by Steven Rhinesmith. Canadian Bureau for International Education, Ottawa Canada. Describes 10 steps of typical cultural adjustment.

Behavior-altering parasites (neuroparasitology):
- "Parasite makes mice lose fear of cats permanently" (18 September 2013), by Eliot Barford, *Nature: News*.
- "Parasitic Puppeteers Begin To Yield Their Secrets" (Jan 17, 2014), *Science Journal* by Elizabeth Pennisie. Short online description of this new field of parasitic influence.

- *Parasite Rex: Inside the Bizarre World of Nature's Most Dangerous Creatures* (2001) by Carl Zimmer. Excellent summary book for non-professionals.
- "Suicidal Crickets, Zombie Roaches and Other Parasite Tales" (March 2014). Presented by Ed Young in the online video series *Ted Talks*.
- *This Is Your Brain on Parasites: How Tiny Creatures Manipulate Our Behavior and Shape Society* (2017) by Kathleen McAuliffe. Written for laypeople.

Reading for professionals

- *Host Manipulation by Parasites* (2012), edited by David Hughes, Jacques Brodeur, and Frederic Thomas. Oxford University Press. Excellent summary of this new field.
- "The Life of a Dead Ant: The Expression of an Adaptive Extended Phenotype" (Sept 2009), *The American Naturalist*, by Sandra B. Andersen et al. Describes the ability of a fungus to control ants, and gives other examples.
- "Mice Infected with Low-Virulence Strains of Toxoplasma gondii Lose Their Innate Aversion to Cat Urine, Even after Extensive Parasite Clearance" (September 18, 2013), by Wendy Marie Ingram, et al., *PLoS One*. A more in-depth article for professionals.

Section 2

Making a Difference

Chapter 5

Treating Ribosomal Voices

In the last chapter we found that a fungus causes ribosomal voices. We described two different approaches for getting rid of them: one on a per-voice basis by healing prenatal trauma, the other on a global basis by making people immune to the fungus. But in engineering terms, these were 'prototype' products. They demonstrated that the techniques (and models) actually worked, but they were neither easy nor painless to use – far from it. They needed well-trained therapists to guide clients, and clients who could follow directions while facing severe emotional and physical trauma.

What were clearly needed were simpler, more effective methods for eliminating ribosomal voices. This chapter is about that search, with the details of how our psychobiology techniques actually worked and how they evolved. We eventually succeeded in two ways: inventing a technique that easily and painlessly gets rid of individual voices; and improving our fungal immunity regression technique, which eliminated all ribosomal voices simultaneously.

We'll end this chapter by looking at different groups of people who can benefit from eliminating ribosomal voices: typical therapy clients; sane people who only hear voices; and people suffering with the severe symptoms of schizophrenia.

In the next chapter, we'll also look at the safety issues and tradeoffs involved with these techniques, and the implications for clients working with therapists or doing self-help. In chapter 7 we'll look at other diseases that can cause a 'noisy' mind. And in chapter 8 we'll discuss our current work on a simpler psycho-immunity approach for getting rid of the fungal disease, one potentially more useful for severe schizophrenia as it also gives the person a continuous feeling of safety.

Psycho-immunology: using regression to eliminate a fungal disease

In chapter 3, we introduced the Silent Mind Technique, but didn't explain how a regression technique that healed prenatal trauma could make someone immune to a subcellular fungal infection. So let's take a look. To do this, we have to cover some subcellular biology that can be experienced during regression but isn't found in biology textbooks, partly because it is tough to observe with current technology, but mostly because no one suspects that there is something important happening there to observe. (So feel free to treat this next part as simply hypothetical, although techniques based on this model actually work, making our models very useful for researchers who are developing new techniques.)

The primordial germ cells (the precursor to egg or sperm cells) first form inside the parental zygote's primary cell, slightly after the parent implants into the grandmother's womb. Inside the parent's primary cell are 7 paired, extremely tiny block-like structures that contain the core awareness of the cell's organelle system, with their multi-celled extension being the triune brains (the body, heart, mind, etc.). When it is time to make a primordial germ cell, the parent buds off new 'kid' blocks, and they eventually leave the primary cell on their way to the area of the zygote that corresponds to the ovary (or testes).

Just after these kid blocks form, they float around separately from each other. Then they enter into parasitic bacteria, like going in a balloon. (This bacterial problem is common in the general population.) We named these balloon-like structures 'pre-organelles'. Soon the blocks start to recombine in a sequence we called 'coalescence'. In 2004 we'd discovered that the mind chatter would go away if one healed trauma in the little bacterial balloon that held the body brain awareness. The critical moment was just after it linked up with the little balloon that held the perineum awareness, but before it linked up with the little balloon that held the heart brain awareness, as shown in figure 5.1. (For more detail about the coalescence event, see *Peak States of Consciousness*, volume 1.) We knew healing this event would usually eliminate the voices, but we didn't know why.

By 2008 we had figured out that we were trying to get rid of free-floating fungus in that body pre-organelle. The next key piece came during a summer-time training in Denmark. Four of the research team members and myself were quietly sitting at an outdoor lunch table, all of us regressed to the same prenatal moment while we tried to figure out what we were missing. Suddenly I sensed the step we'd overlooked and spontaneously said in a loud voice a word that matched what I was feeling. My colleagues all jumped, and the little octopus-looking fungi suddenly vanished out of the precellular organelles they were observing. This command or directive word is something we call a Gaia command – it is a verbal translation of what the cell is supposed to do at that moment. (Unfortunately, working with just that one word alone has unfortunate side effects – it can make a person feel extreme pain in the present as they feel lumps coming out of their body. Hence we have not included it in this book.) It wasn't until the fall of 2011 that we got all the steps for this event (making treatment more reliable) and really understood what needed to happen.

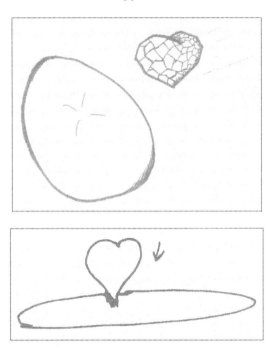

Figure 5.1: The coalescence event just before the body and the heart pre-organelles combine. The heart structure resembles a turnip or stylized heart; the body structure resembles a fat pancake. Upper: the heart approaching the body. Lower: the heart entering the body.

In this particular moment of development, it was possible to first induce the pre-organelle into secreting a chemical that dissolves the fungus. When the octopus-like fungal organisms are dead and mostly dissolved (in the regression), the cell could then excrete the remains. Once the pre-organelle cell was cleared of these remains – like cleaning out a plugged toilet - the body stopped assuming that this fungus was supposed to be there. In the present, it would suddenly recognize the fungus as foreign and quickly destroy it. The body's speed is remarkable – the mind would go silent in the present while the client was still finishing healing the key step in the past.

More background: psycho-immunology

Over the decades, based on the phenomenon of spontaneous, placebo effect, and emotional release work cures, many have theorized that people were somehow responsible for their diseases. The entire field of psycho-immunology (now usually called psychoneuroimmunology) was based on this idea, that we were not victims but rather somehow participating in our illnesses. But the underlying biology was not understood and frustratingly there were no repeatable, reliable techniques to demonstrate this hypothesis.

This situation has now changed with the recent advent of effective trauma techniques, an understanding of prenatal developmental stages, and recognition of problems and diseases in the primary cell. The body may or may not want the symptoms, damage or death that diseases cause – but it can't break its own need for the problem without help. As we've shown with the borg fungus, one approach for inducing disease immunity using trauma therapy is to eliminate the body's mistaken conviction that the disease organisms are supposed to be present. However, as they say, "one shoe does not fit all". In our experience with other diseases, the body has problems identifying friend from foe for a variety of different reasons. Amazingly, once those reasons are gone, the disease is *immediately* destroyed.

At this point, astute readers are probably saying, "Whoa, wait a minute! What do you mean the pre-organelle cell in the past now gets rid of the fungus? The past is fixed!" This is a natural assumption for people outside the field of trauma therapy. True, when a trauma is fully healed, the client suddenly feels calm and no longer cares about the event, no matter how painful it had been up to then. We can all accept that and be grateful that a new generation of extremely effective trauma techniques now exists. However, what we see using *any* trauma technique goes beyond that. After a client *fully* eliminates a past trauma, they now have two pasts: the one they remember, and the new one they can now experience when they actually put their attention back into that past moment. This really bizarre effect is especially observable in regression; in that past moment, they now act in new ways to the outer circumstances.

We don't go into the theory with clients – we simply regress them to the relevant moment using a visualization with words and music, and have them heal every sensation and emotion they feel until they are calm and peaceful. Interestingly, an important step in the process just described is to heal what therapists call 'generational trauma' – the same phenomenon that biologists call 'inherited epigenetic damage'. The ability to kill and eject the fungus is often blocked by traumatic experiences from our ancestors; otherwise, these steps would have just been done automatically and we would never have gotten the problem in the first place.

This process can take anywhere from an hour to up to nine hours under the guidance of a trauma therapist. Both the primordial germ cell in the mother and the one in the father need to be healed. This can be a fascinating experience; first one side of the head goes silent as one of the primordial germ cells is healed, and then the other side goes silent when the other one is finished. And the tribal block problem also vanishes - there are no longer any emotional tones coming in the navel when you think about what you want to do, and you lose your reaction to people from different cultures or races. Unfortunately, many clients report that they still have their attraction to people with particular emotional tones. Those associational ribosomes still exit, but they don't have the 'voices' crystals in them anymore.

However, I was still unsatisfied with the ease and speed of that treatment, especially for schizophrenic client populations. In the next sections we'll look at how we worked to solve that problem.

More background: immunity to all diseases

We've written several textbooks that outline some of the underlying prenatal developmental event data and various techniques we've developed for specific diseases. In particular, the *Subcellular Psychobiology Diagnosis Handbook*, and *Peak States of Consciousness* Volumes 1 and 2 are useful for research work in psycho-immunology. We spend much of our time trying to figure out the link between diseases of unknown etiology (for example, autism or diabetes), their cause in the primary cell, and treatments based on developmental event trauma.

Of far more interest to us is that our models predict that it is possible to eliminate an entire class of diseases all at once with one process, such as eliminating all fungal species, or all harmful bacterial species, or all viral species, or all types of prions. Especially with the advent of antibiotic-resistant diseases and the possibility of global viral pandemics, this critically important area is where the majority of our research time is spent.

Speaking personally, our model also predicts that these same global disease treatments will also make fundamental changes in human consciousness, which is really why my team continues to work on these problems in spite of the suffering and risks involved in the research.

The Body Association Technique™: A simple, painless way to eliminate a ribosomal voice

As we've seen, regression techniques have drawbacks, especially for clients who have difficulty in facing pain or following directions. We needed another approach, ideally something simple and pain-free that anyone could use. This search dragged on for many years, but I was not willing to publish until we'd solved this problem.

Back in 1995, I'd noticed while getting rid of my own voices that I could do it without actually healing the prenatal trauma. I would focus my attention on my mom's feeling side by side with my survival feeling, and send love at the junction between them. And poof, they would split apart and the voice would vanish. I tried teaching this to others but with very mixed success. It wasn't until 2004 or so that we realized what I'd been doing - that old technique was splitting the mRNA string that held the ribosomal voice from the ribosome with the survival feeling.

During the 2000s, I was also working with the dedicated, amazing drug and alcohol therapist Matt Fox, trying to find a treatment for addiction using our new subcellular and regression psychobiology approach. Over years, we came to find out that many addictions are due to body associations. Matt came up with a technique that could get rid of those associations, but it was rather complicated and needed a therapist to guide the client. But it did work, and so allowed us to verify our hypothesis about addictive cravings and withdrawal. (For more on this, see our upcoming book on addictions.)

But in the back of my mind I was constantly thinking about easier ways to eliminate body associations. Looking back, I almost solved it in 2009 with a technique similar to what we have now, but it only worked for some people. It wasn't until 2012, while training students in Ashland, Oregon that I suddenly thought of a simple modification that might improve the technique. I tested the idea on the spot, and it was amazing! Anyone could do it, it had no side effects, and it was exactly what I'd been looking for to treat addictions and other irrational associations. Moments like that don't come often in research; I can't help but smile as I think back to that day and those students.

But as we'd seen, a ribosomal voice is also from a body association. And this technique turned out to be absolutely perfect for getting rid of them. In just minutes, a voice could be painlessly and permanently eliminated by just about anyone.

How? Well, I have a person put their hands face up in a slightly cupped position. Then I have them imagine that they have a crumpled bag, like a ball, held in their hand. This imaginary bag would then radiate the emotional tone of the voice. Then the person would tap on the back of their hand that was holding the imaginary bag for about 1-2 minutes, and the bag would either fly up or melt away in their hand. This latter effect could be quite a surprise to the person, as this happens without their will or control. (See Appendix D for detailed steps with illustrations.)

This trick is elegantly simple, as it relies on the fact that sensations from one's physical body are superimposed on sensations from the primary cell. To the body, the upwardly cupped hand *feels* like the endoplasmic reticulum (ER) membrane with a pore in it, as if your hand were the pore's rim. The crumpled bag feels like a ribosome that radiates the sensation it contains (in this case the voice's emotional tone that came from the mother during the fetal injury moment). By holding out your hand while imagining a bag with the target emotional tone, you unconsciously sort through all the stuck ribosomes in the ER to find the right one.

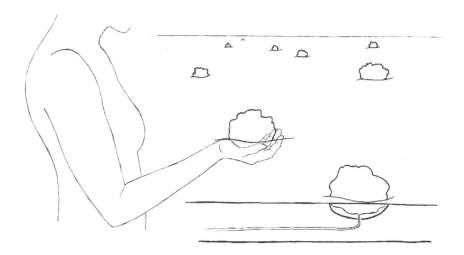

Figure 5.2: To the body consciousness, it feels like it has a hand holding each ribosome imbedded in a pore in its rough endoplasmic reticulum membrane. (The rough ER is shown in a cutaway view; each ribosome also has an mRNA string connecting it to a stuck gene in the nucleus.)

The second half of the trick involves meridian therapy. EFT, the most famous of these techniques, has people focus on an emotional tone while tapping on Chinese acupuncture points. A few years earlier we'd realized that we could get similar results by just tapping on the back of the hand at what's called the 9-gamut point. The reason many people didn't realize this was possible was because there was a time delay involved. It usually took between one and two minutes for any change to happen. This is because tapping on this point repairs the damaged histone proteins covering a stuck gene. No symptoms would change until the histone damage was repaired enough to release the stuck mRNA string attached to the gene – then poof, the mRNA string would let go, the ribosome attached to it would pop out of the ER's pore, and one would feel the ribosome (the crumpled bag) popping out of the hand (or partially melt away if there were more than one stuck gene involved).

This body association technique is incredibly useful, painless and fast, taking only about 2 minutes per voice. And as we've pointed out, many people who have a ribosomal voice problem just need only one to three eliminated to make a world of difference in their lives. And of course, one can keep using the technique to get a fully silent mind (given that one doesn't keep making new ones) by noticing and eliminate any voices that come into awareness. As an added bonus, it also gets rid of the irrational sexual attractions to people with certain emotional tones.

What are its drawbacks? First, people may get *new* voices that also need to be treated and eliminated; this is triggered by their loneliness and need to have 'people' in their lives. They still had 'empty' ribosomes ready for a voice, but fortunately their supply is very finite. While potentially disruptive or annoying, it is simple to repeat the body association process. Secondly, everyone hears voices, but people who've lost their mute control generally had a trauma experience that they felt was somehow life threatening. That trauma won't go away with the voices, and may need to be dealt with. And lastly, this technique does *not* get rid of the underlying borg fungus infection with all its other issues (such as the tribal block problem).

Tip for therapists:
If you want to find out if their problem is really due to ribosomal voices, we recommend you first try the body association technique on the worst voice(s). This simple, fast technique will let you quickly decide if anything more needs to be done, or whether their issue is actually due to ribosomal voices or not. If so, you can then decide if you also want to use the more difficult and slow Silent Mind Technique regression (or the new one coming online in late 2017). Of course, there are other good reasons besides eliminating ribosomal voices to want to get rid of the fungus, such as tribal block, cross-cultural issues, etc.

Who can be helped with ribosomal voice techniques?

To help the reader, let's review the various groups of clients we've mentioned who can benefit from eliminating their ribosomal voices or the borg fungus. (For in-depth diagnostic criteria see the *Subcellular Psychobiology Diagnosis Handbook*.) Voice hearers are somewhere between 5 and 15% of the general population, which means there are a *lot* of people who can obviously be helped with just a voice treatment. Below, we've ordered all of the problems resulting from the borg fungus in the approximate frequency that we see them as private practice clients. For now we'll exclude the obviously mentally ill until the next section. Of course, as we've seen virtually *everyone* has background thoughts or tribal block influences from the borg infection and could benefit from treatment – they just don't know it.

Interpersonal issues: These problems are often diagnosed as transference or counter-transference and are caused by 'cording' via the borg fungus. In rare cases, we see the more extreme case of 'curses' causing physical pain and other symptoms. The choice of technique depends on the therapist and what the client is willing to feel in the way of discomfort. The Distant Personality Release technique is usually adequate on a problem-by-problem basis, but getting rid of the underlying fungal infection can be more efficient in terms of time if they have a number of these issues.

Emotional issues: Occasionally the therapist assumes the client has an emotional issue when it is actually a voice problem (or in addition to their emotional issue). The voices problem can show up in counter-intuitive ways because people assume the voice is their own. For example, the client comes in with an issue, say anxiety, but it is because they have an anxious voice, but don't actually feel anxious themselves. The simple body association technique is ideal.

Racing/intrusive thoughts: People whose ribosomal voices are muted so they don't 'hear voices' will experienced them as 'background thoughts'. In some cases, these thoughts can still be experienced as a problem, especially in the case of racing or intrusive thoughts that they can't stop. In other cases, the content of the thoughts is what bothers the client. Although there can be other causes for this problem (see the next chapter), typically this can be easily treated with the body association technique.

Meditators/personal growth clients: These people often want the silent mind state to make their meditation easier. They are usually not interested in the other problems from the borg infection. The body association technique is usually adequate, although they may want to simply experience the borg fungus immunity technique.

Hearing voices clients: These are the people who clearly hear voices but are otherwise completely normal. This includes people whose voices can range from positive or helpful to extremely negative. The body association technique is usually adequate for them, but getting rid of the borg fungus can make it simpler as the voices go all at once, and new ones won't appear.

Sexual addictions: The client might have a sexual addiction, which can usually be treated by eliminating the body associations driving it. This is by far the most common mechanism, although there are other possible causes – for more on this, we refer you to our book on addictions.

Multicultural-issue clients: These people either have strong reactions to other races or cultures, are terrified of being in a new culture, or reject the culture they used to be a part of. The best solution is to make them immune to the borg fungus.

Channeling or possessed clients: These clients have been simple to help in our limited experience. Their problems were due to only one or two ribosomal voices, so the body association technique was ideal. (Note that after their problem is gone, some clients may also need help healing any fear or revulsion they had from having the experience.)

Struggle with altruistic goals: In our experience, this problem occurs most frequently in highly functional people as they are generally willing to resist the tribal block influence more than any other group. They seldom have an issue with voices, and rarely need any other therapy. Hence, the 'one issue at a time' tribal block technique is usually ideal.

However, in our experience there are also some clients who don't want treatment, and the therapist has to be ready to accept this. First, one group includes people whose culture supports having voices. For example, one client I saw was from Africa. In his particular culture, it was considered positive to hear the voices of ancestors or other tribal members. Hence, even though his voices were causing problems for him and his Canadian partner, he refused to consider getting rid of them. Secondly are people who would feel lonely or abandoned without their voices. For example, one client I saw really enjoyed one of her voices because it felt so friendly and would tell her jokes. If they do choose to get their voices eliminated, they will need to have help in making the adjustment to life without this problem.

Summary table of our relevant therapy techniques and their uses

Technique	Use	Speed / risk	Where found
Body Association Technique™, rev 2.0[1]	Eliminates individual ribosomal voice	Very fast and effective / minimal risk; a few potential adjustment issues	Appendix D
Distant Personality Release™ (DPR)	Eliminates individual cord or curse	Fast and effective / minimal risk; a few possible problems	*The Basic Whole-Hearted Healing Manual,* pp 84, 195.
Tribal Block Technique™, rev 1.7	Eliminates individual tribal block issue	Fast and effective / minimal risk; some cautions	Appendix E
Silent Mind Technique™ (SMT), rev 2.3[2,3]	Permanently eliminates *all* voices, cords, curses, & tribal block issues	Slow (2-9 hrs) / some potential trauma healing issues	Proprietary - taught in therapist courses
'Listening to Silence' peak state process	Profound inner silence – does *not* eliminate borg fungus	Difficult / state unstable with process in this book	Pg. 45

Note 1: This versatile technique has to be used in a specific way to eliminate voices.
Note 2: This applies only to the ribosomal voices type.
Note 3: For advertising purposes, SMT is used as an umbrella term for our various voice-related treatments.

How successful is this for treating schizophrenia?

What percentage of people diagnosed with schizophrenia return to normal after eliminating ribosomal voices or the borg fungus with our current processes? What we're really interested in here is how many people with an obvious mental illness can be helped with these treatments. (We exclude here the mentally well 'voice hearers' covered in the previous section.)

The answer is we simply don't know, as we have not had the opportunity to do any large-scale tests with our current techniques. But based on feedback from therapists we've trained, we *guess* that roughly 20% of the obviously mentally ill people who also hear voices can be restored to health by these techniques. Fortunately, this is still a huge number of people when one remembers that 1% of the human race has a schizophrenia diagnosis.

Why so (relatively) few? First of all, about 30% of the people diagnosed with schizophrenia *don't* hear voices (Hoffman, Yale News, 2001). Thus, a voices treatment would usually not make any difference to them. Secondly, the current diagnosis of schizophrenia is made up of different collections of symptoms, but this does *not* mean we're seeing symptoms from just one disease. Thus some may have a mental illness problem with ribosomal voices as a second, unrelated issue. Knowing which disease is causing the symptoms matters because the treatments are usually totally different. Third, there are less common types of voices that the client might have (see chapter 7).

So which schizophrenics can we help? In general, it comes down to three groups:

- People whose symptoms of mental illness are in response to the verbal *content* (and emotional tone) of their voices. In other words, they retreat from reality or act delusional because they are trying to resist what they believe is part of themselves, the voices they hear. For example, paranoia (F20.0) or catatonia (F20.2) might be good candidates for treatment (although paranoia can also be caused by other problems.)
- People whose symptoms of mental illness are from the *torture* of continuous, loud voices in their mind. Like prisoners being tortured, they retreat from reality due to sleep loss and the non-stop noise. These people also display problems interacting with the outer world while the loud voices are present. For example, 'acute and transient psychotic disorders' (F23) might be caused by this.
- People whose symptoms are due to the life-threatening *trauma* that triggered the inability to mute their internal voices. (This threat is in their perception, not necessarily in objective reality.) What can happen is that the voices cause positive feedback – the presence of voices keeps the underlying trauma triggered, which keeps the voices un-muted, and so on, keeping the cycle going. Or the trauma is in itself causing strange behavior, especially when it is forgotten or suppressed. For example, schizotypal disorders (F21) might be caused this way.

Obviously, it can be difficult to sort out if the voices are causing symptoms of mental illness, or is the mental illness caused by something else entirely and the voices are simply an added, unrelated burden. What is the therapist to do? At the present time, we suggest simply trying to work with your client and see if you can help them identify any voices that are causing them problems, and start from there. This can be tricky in cases where the person felt uncomfortable or distraught without realizing that they were hearing a very negative voice – they were simply suppressing or ignoring it, but noticing in the background the emotional tone of the voice, or feeling the symptoms of their suppression, or both.

Given all this, why aren't all voice hearers showing signs of mental illness? There are several reasons:

- The content and emotional tone of the voices can really matter as to a person's response. People dealing with voices that feel like the essence of evil or of hating, raging maniacs will have a harder time staying stable than people who have voices that cheerfully tell jokes and give friendly encouragement.
- How a person responds to crisis and stress can really vary. Some people fall apart from relatively mild problems, while others stay stable living in horrific situations.
- The person might not have a predisposition or pre-existing condition – in this case, a susceptibility to or dormant disease process, be it subcellular or extracellular, that causes a particular mental illness symptom.

More background: the number of voices in a person

The typical, non-patient person has an average of approximately 15 ribosomal voices, with a standard deviation of about 5 voices. The difference between an average person and a person diagnosed with schizophrenia is usually in the severity and negativity of the voices, not their absolute number; although we've seen that some members of the patient group can have a significantly higher number of voices than the non-patient population.

In this book we've identified one of the most common problems in humanity, ribosomal voices, but in our research into subcellular psychobiology we've seen *many* different diseases or structural problems that can affect one's mental state. And this does not even include diseases (parasites, bacteria and fungus) that one can see in the gut or body that also have a psychological effect.

I want to end this section by emphasizing that generations of hard working, dedicated physicians, psychologists, and laypeople have done their absolute best to try and make diagnostic categories, hoping it would help researchers find causes and treatments for the suffering that these mentally ill people experience. Unfortunately, progress was limited because they didn't realize that subcellular diseases exist that can cause the psychological symptoms of mental illness. Hopefully in the next few decades more of these subcellular diseases will be identified and psychological or drug-based treatments will be created.

What about other mental disorders?

What about other mental disorders that include voices? In my experience, they are usually two totally unrelated problems that are lumped together. When we eliminate the ribosomal voices (which often helps a great deal of the client's distress), the other symptoms still remain.

How common is this combination of independent problems? Honig et al. (1998) says around 25% of affective psychosis patients hear voices. Using the ICD-10 categories (the International Statistical Classification of Diseases and Related Health Problems), we see the following subcategories of mood (affective) disorders that potentially include voices.

- Mania with psychotic symptoms (F30.2).
- Bipolar affective disorder, current episode manic with psychotic symptoms (F31.2).
- Bipolar affective disorder, current episode severe depression with psychotic symptoms (F31.5).
- Severe depressive episode with psychotic symptoms (F32.3).
- Recurrent depressive disorder, current episode severe with psychotic symptoms (F33.3).

For example, in our experience bipolar disorder is a completely unrelated disease to voices. So is depression (although in some cases it is the voices that are depressed and the client assumes they are too; or their presence drives the client into feeling depressed).

Similarly, Honig et al. says about 80% of dissociative (conversion) disorders also include voices. Note that there are two categories directly relevant to a ribosomal voice treatment.

- Dissociative stupor (F44.2). There is a possibility this problem is triggered by successful suppression of suddenly activated voices.
- Trance and possession disorders (F44.3). This case we covered in the previous section, where removing ribosomal voices does eliminate the problem.

Pay for results

So, how do you find a therapist who can do these techniques? You can always take this book to your therapist or into your local clinic or health center and ask them to do the process with you. If they are unfamiliar with the technique, relatively fast training is available for trauma therapists. If your health practitioner does not use trauma therapies, then their training might take a bit longer.

Fortunately, our 'Silent Mind Technique' works fairly well, and for years we've taught it to therapists all over the world. One of the things that makes these therapists stand out from others is that they all work on a 'pay for results' basis. What does this mean? If your voices problem didn't go away after treatment, or came back and they can't fix it, there is no fee. Therapists trained by us will have you sign an agreement with you on the results you both expect from treatment. If those results don't happen, then you don't pay (or get a refund, if that was the contract agreement).

We have our therapists do this for a lot of reasons. First, the 'golden rule' – do unto others as you would have them do unto you. After all, if it doesn't work, why should you pay? How do you feel when your plumber or car mechanic charges you but nothing got fixed? Secondly, many people who are desperately in need of help don't have much money. If they work with a therapist who wastes their precious cash but doesn't give them the service they were expecting, they don't have money left to get help elsewhere. Third, it makes legitimate therapists, who use state-of-the-art techniques that really work stand out. And finally, if a therapist is only paid for doing a good job, pretty soon they become really, really good at it, or they quit. This makes sure that you don't get financially penalized if your therapist is unskilled or just doesn't really have any talent for the work.

How does this 'pay for results' work from the therapist viewpoint? Well, first of all, the techniques work pretty well. So your therapist expects most clients to get success, and so he'll get paid by most of them. But say it doesn't work for you. These therapists set their standard price a bit higher to account for the clients who don't work out. This is exactly what your car dealer or local grocer does, and it is normal in a lot of industries. (See Appendix A for a sample contract.)

Finally, this helps you separate out legitimate, trained therapists from unscrupulous people who are willing to promise you anything as long as they get paid. How? Get a charge for results contract first and pay them after the agreed upon changes are met. With the Silent Mind Technique, the results will happen right in their office.

Meet the team - Steve and Jessie Hsu

Steve writes: "What is the meaning of life? Is there a God? Why is there so much suffering in the world? These were the questions that haunted me in my younger years and helped lay the foundation as I matriculate through life. Looking back it's unmistakable that there seemed to be an invisible force taking care of me and gently guiding me through twists and turns. As I map out my accumulated insights and understanding into "who I am", "why I am here", and this thing we call "life", those haunting questions slowly dissolved somehow, like a shift in perspective that made them irrelevant.

"Looking around it's not difficult to suspect something is deeply wrong with the world, or more precisely the human species that created this world. But what? There are numerous philosophical proposals, such as, we harm each other because we don't feel we are all one, or how can we create peace in the world when we can't find peace in ourselves. These are really challenging issues. Can we solve this problem? Is it even possible? It seems to me that religion, philosophy, psychology, and such are trying to solve the same problem. If it's possible to create lasting change in a person to have deep inner peace, if it's possible to feel we are all members of a one loving family, not mentally, but at the visceral level, there just might be hope for humanity and life on earth. Silencing the voices is a good start."

Key Points

- It is possible to induce immunity to a pathogen by using psychological techniques that heal early key developmental events.
- During the formation of the primordial germ cell is the 'coalescence' developmental event. Healing part of it can induce fungal immunity.
- Biologists have not yet looked for the tiny, subcellular coalescence event; but regression by clients to the event is simple.
- All trauma-healing techniques have potential problems, so clients need to read and sign a disclosure form to understand the tradeoffs and risks.

- Regression to certain prenatal events can also have safety issues. When developing a new technique, testing is required to ensure safety.
- Offering psychological services on a 'pay for results' basis is both ethical and helps avoid the problem of unscrupulous people offering treatments that do not work or are harmful.
- The Body Association Technique™ can be used to easily, painlessly, and safely eliminate individual ribosomal voices. However, some people will be uncomfortable when their voices vanish, or if new voices appear later.
- Most voice hearers can have their voices permanently removed by using psychological techniques that either eliminate subcellular ribosomes or make the person immune to the borg fungus.
- The Silent Mind Technique™ uses a psycho-immunology process that eliminates the borg fungus, and so gets rid all symptoms that are caused by the fungus (ribosomal voices, cords, tribal block, etc.)
- 1% of the general population is diagnosed with schizophrenia. Of this group, somewhere between 70% and 80% also hear voices.
- Only some people with schizophrenia can be treated successfully by eliminating ribosomal voices. Others have symptoms from unrelated causes. The percentage that is healed by eliminating ribosomal voices (using current techniques) is uncertain due to lack of testing.
- People with affective psychosis and dissociative disorders can sometimes have voices, but the voices are usually a separate issue. However, the trance and possession disorder is generally due to ribosomal voices.

Suggested Reading

Psychoeuroimmunology:
- "Epigenetics, psychoneuroimmunology, and subcellular psychobiology" (2014) by Grant McFetridge on www.PeakStates.com
- "The Biology of Epigenetic Trauma" (2016) by Grant McFetridge on www.PeakStates.com
- *Peak States of Consciousness*, Volume 2 (2008), by Grant McFetridge. See chapter 4 for details on the problem of epigenetically inhibited gene expression. See Chapter 8 and Appendix F for developmental events relevant to psycho-immunology.

Pay for results:

- *Subcellular Psychobiology Diagnosis Handbook* (2014), by Grant McFetridge. See chapter 3 and appendices 2 and 10.

Safety issues with regression and trauma therapy:

- *Peak States of Consciousness, Volume 2* (2008), by Grant McFetridge and Wes Geitz. See Appendix A. (Chapters 10 and 17 also contains in-depth information on Gaia commands.)
- *Subcellular Psychobiology Diagnosis Handbook* (2014), by Grant McFetridge. See chapter 6.

Voices in patient versus non-patient groups:

- "Auditory hallucinations: a comparison between patients and nonpatients" (1998), Honig A., Romme M. A. J., Ensink B. J., Escher S. D. M. A. C., Pennings M. H. A., deVries M. W., *Journal of Nervous and Mental Disease*, 186(10), 646–651.

Relevant therapies:

- "Clinical benefits of Peak States Therapies" in *Positive Health Magazine*, Sept. 2007, Issue 139, www.PositiveHealth.com.
- *The Whole-Hearted Healing Workbook* (2013) by Paula Courteau. Projection, regression, and subcellular treatments for laypeople.
- *The Basic Whole-Hearted Healing Manual* (2004) by Grant McFetridge Ph.D. Contains DPR, regression, and other techniques. Written for professionals.
- *The EFT Manual*, 6th edition, by Gary Craig. Excellent tutorial on the EFT meridian therapy for trauma. Written for laypeople.

Chapter 6

Safety Issues and Side Effects

After what you've read in the previous chapter, you might be saying to yourself "Sign me up!" And for most people this would be a great choice with a problem-free outcome, a bit like taking your car into the dealership for repair. However, what many laypeople don't realize is that there are tradeoffs even with ordinary psychological techniques. And the techniques in this book are far more powerful than typical talk therapy – these affect the very insides of your cells.

In previous chapters we focused on what can go right. In this chapter we'll look at what can go wrong. We'll cover some of the obvious and, at least to laypeople, far less obvious problems – and solutions – that one might encounter using these techniques. This chapter is also valuable for therapists or physicians whose training may not have included extensive work with trauma or regression therapies.

We'll also briefly look at how clients taking antipsychotic medication need to be handled differently, with guidance, caution and forethought when using these psychobiological techniques.

Trauma therapies: risks and informed consent

Let's first look at some of the standard risks that can occur using *any* trauma technique on the usual run of client issues. (This discussion is just to give you general background. The current Silent Mind Technique is more specialized than standard trauma therapy, and we'll look at its issues in more detail in the next section.)

- During treatment, you will feel worse before you start to feel better.
- You *will* encounter uncomfortable or unfamiliar emotional pain (in that you may feel anger, sadness, guilt, grief, loss, frustration, etc.)

as well as physical discomforts or pains (such as nausea, suffocation, aches, or other pain).

- If you do not fully heal during a treatment, your symptoms will persist for a time, until those memories re-submerge and leave your awareness or you return for your next session.
- If you stop in the middle of treatment, you will usually feel worse than when you started.
- A few unlucky people can trigger pain that just won't stop without a specific intervention.
- Some people will find that their change is unstable, and will require another session.
- Not all problems or issues can be helped.
- Some issues will be worse after treatment.

As odd as it sounds to therapists, the biggest surprise many laypeople have is that trauma therapy is often emotionally and physically painful. How much and how long depends on your issue and the particular techniques you need. For example, using meridian ('tapping') therapies, any pain is *usually* both minimal and brief. But even using those therapies you can encounter some pretty painful experiences; and other therapies can be far worse. However, if you realize it is like going to the dentist, just something that hurts for a bit but needs to be done, you'll have the right mindset for doing therapy. Unfortunately, in some cases the therapy won't work at all, or you can finish therapy feeling worse than you started. Although this is getting more uncommon as therapists switch to the newer generation of techniques, it *can* still happen. You have to decide if the risk of getting better versus the (unlikely) possibly of getting worse is worth it to you.

Therapists are required by law (in most countries) to have you read and sign an informed consent form. This covers the usual and the unexpected issues that can arise in therapy. You should be concerned if your therapist has not given you one to read! For a copy of the one our Institute uses, see Appendix C.

For more on potential problems with trauma and regression therapies, we suggest reading the references at the end of this chapter.

Risks with the Body Association Technique

Up to this point, we've just been talking about trauma therapy for the usual run of client issues. By contrast, as you've read in the previous chapter, our Body Association Technique is *not* a trauma therapy. Instead, it interacts directly with subcellular structures, and thankfully it is *both* painless and reliable for the type of problems it was designed to treat. After 5 years and many hundreds of clients, we've seen no adverse or unexpected side effects from using this technique. In fact, it is remarkably robust and problem free.

However, issues can arise after a *successful* treatment. First, getting rid of some or all their voices can make the client suddenly and unexpectedly feel lonely. This can be like walking through your grade school after everyone has left for summer vacation. For some this loneliness won't occur, for some it is mild and can be ignored, but in some people it can be sudden and severe. This problem can have various causes. The most likely is called 'soul loss'. Less frequently, it can be caused by simple biographical trauma, or due to 'holes'. (See the *Whole-Hearted Healing Workbook* for details). In all three cases, simple tapping with EFT or another meridian therapy almost always eliminates this feeling.

Another problem can sometimes occur also after a successful treatment. In this case, the client finishes the session feeling great. Later, they interact with someone and suddenly notice a new voice. More commonly they interact and suddenly feel worse, usually with a heavy or depressed feeling, but don't notice a new voice. What has happened in this latter case is that they now have a new 'voice' but its feeling and words are so unpleasant they instantly suppressed it from awareness. This can be tricky to spot, as it happens suddenly and the person may not notice the new voice unless their attention is directed to look for it. (Of course, it may be a totally unrelated problem – just ordinary issues with the other person.) Once this new voice is noticed, simply repeating the body association technique quickly solves the problem.

Lastly, again after a successful treatment, the irrational sexual attractions the person had will just vanish. This can be a real problem if the person suddenly looses sexual interest in their spouse or partner. There is no way to return the client back to how they were. However, people tend to be attracted to each other for a variety of reasons. In our experience, this problem passes after a while (from days to months) and conjugal relations resume. This is not guaranteed, however – although we haven't yet seen this happen, this might cause a divorce as well as strong confusion and disappointment in both partners.

Risks with the regression Silent Mind Technique

If you are considering using the current revision 2.3 version of the Silent Mind Technique (that uses regression) to make yourself immune to the borg fungus, what are some of the potential issues?

A regression technique that targets a specific problem or disorder is a bit analogous to using a drug for a particular illness. Unlike general therapy, after seeing many clients over time, pretty much all of the unexpected issues have already been seen and worked out. Hence, we can teach a course on this technique that just focuses on mastering it and its problems. It is a bit like learning to change your car oil versus learning how to be a mechanic. Of course, people can be amazingly complicated and so it is always a good idea to know a highly trained trauma therapist that can be called in case something unexpected or unusual comes up. Following the car analogy, sometimes the old junker you are working on breaks a bolt as you try to remove the oil filter. So you call up your local mechanic to pass on this problem.

So let's look at some of the potential problems:

Another disorder is present: Assuming a process has already been well tested on typical people, problems can arise if you have another disorder that interferes or interacts badly with the treatment. The most frequent case is an anxiety disorder. In this case, trying to heal may only make their anxiety worse, and will probably mask their ability to sense the trauma feelings they need to heal to get a psycho-immunological effect.

The spouse's reaction: This problem shows up about half the time with couples where only one partner is treated. After successful treatment, the client feels fine but the untreated partner reports that the other now feels distant and separate from them. This is because all the fungal cords are now gone. The simplest fix is to also treat the partner.

Loneliness: After successful treatment, some clients will feel lonely now that they are without their voices. We see this often in people diagnosed with severe mental illness. Treatment for this is the same as with the Body Association Technique.

Sounds seem louder: Once the voices are gone, it is like all of the people in the nightclub you've been sitting in have left. This means other sounds will suddenly seem much louder to you. In general, this is a good thing; but in one case we had, the person now needed to use earplugs at work because the sound of the engines seemed suddenly far louder. In another case, the person's pre-existing tinnitus suddenly seemed louder.

Suicidal feelings: Just as with *any* therapeutic intervention, as a precaution the therapist needs to have been trained to recognize and deal with the problem of suicidal activation. The regression itself is going to bring up intense feelings, and since one of the possible outcomes of a successful treatment is sudden loneliness, the possibility for suicidal activation exists. As far as the Silent Mind Technique is concerned, there are four cases to look at:

1. Someone who has never felt suicidal. Fortunately, we've never seen a client triggered into a suicidal episode. But people are complex, and a therapist should always be on the lookout for this issue.

2. The client had suicidal feelings in the past but not at present. Obviously there is now some risk. This is a judgment call for the therapist, one that depends on the training of the therapist and support available to the client. First, should the therapist work with this client at all? If they do, how long is long enough since the last episode? Most of the therapists we work with don't do this process with someone with a history of suicidal feelings, but they will refer them to those who do. Again, we haven't seen a problem yet, but a lot more cautions should be taken.

3. The client is actively suicidal. We do *not* recommend working with these clients outside of a 24-hour watch facility. The feelings during the regression and afterwards might exacerbate their suicide issue, or in the extreme, cause them to commit suicide. Instead, we recommend the client get suicide intervention and wait until their problem has been in remission for some preset period of time.

4. The client hears a suicidal *voice*, but does *not* have suicidal feelings. We've actually seen this odd case a number of times. Fortunately, treatment is simple. Use the body association technique to eliminate the suicidal voice then re-evaluate the client. Obviously, cases like these have some risk of misdiagnosis, but the therapist is usually able to spot this situation very easily. If they still report suicidal feelings after the voice is gone, treat them as you would any active suicide patient.

Be honest with your therapist; you *don't* want to surprise them in the middle of treatment.

More background: publishing techniques

We're sometimes asked why we don't publish our detailed process steps for healing prenatal developmental events. Obviously, the safety issues above are part of that reason – the lay public can start, encounter pain and suffering that they were not expecting, and get stuck. But from a research perspective, this allows us to continue improving our techniques without worrying about less effective or unexpectedly problematic 'legacy' processes. It also allows us to do more testing - therapists who are trained by us give us feedback if unusual problems arise as more and more people use the processes; and our clinic staff can assist the therapist and client if needed.

Books like this have to draw a fine line – we want this material to be educational and useful for laypeople, therapists and researchers, but not so detailed that laypeople might be tempted to experiment. However, there are exceptions. We do publish many of our safe *non*-regression techniques after they've had many years of testing. In fact, two of them can be found in this book's appendices.

Clients using antipsychotic medications

If you are currently using antipsychotic medication, and after treatment you suddenly feel well, do *not* stop taking your medication.

This is for a number of reasons. The most important – your medication may be masking another psychiatric problem besides ribosomal voices. Going off the drugs may restart a mental illness issue that was hidden by the drugs. Secondly, some of these drugs have nasty side effects if you abruptly stop taking them.

What to do if you are the therapist? First, standard therapist training is not adequate for working with this client group - you need training and practice in how to interact with people with severe mental illness who are taking antipsychotics. Second, the therapist needs to work with the client's physician before, during, and after treatment. The temptation to just quit medication will be strong with some clients – so the therapist should also confirm that the client has an appointment with the physician to review medication use after the client has finished the silent mind process.

Remember, people are like old beat up cars – they can have a lot of problems!

Client suitability evaluation checklist

What constitutes an acceptable client depends on the training of the therapist and the facilities available for the client. The guidelines below are designed for *private practice therapists* in a typical office setting, and *not* for a hospital with constant care facilities or in a 24-hour suicide watch facility. (In that case, many of these restrictions no longer apply.)

The client IS an ideal candidate:
- *Rational:* The client is aware that they have a problem with 'mind chatter' or 'voices'. The client can rationally discuss their problem with voices. They have no other significant issues.

- *Time commitment:* The client is willing to commit to multiple therapy sessions and the progressive healing using this approach. Typical treatment time is 1 to 9 hours in total.
- *No complicating factors:* Aside from the voices or the consequences of hearing voices, the client has no other complicating conditions.

The client MAY BE a suitable candidate:

- *Current crisis:* Any current issue needs to be dealt with first.
- *Illegal psychoactive drugs:* They are currently or recently using 'recreational' drugs. The major problem is the possibility that the drugs have activated other, disabling prenatal trauma that might make treatment ineffective. Additionally, there is always a (small) chance that the drugs might help trigger a psychotic break during the treatment period.
- *Psycho-active medication:* They are currently using psycho-active prescription medication. If the client's MD is working with the therapist on drug dosage, this would be OK. Otherwise, they are NOT suitable for this process. This is due to two major problems: 1) only an MD should (and can legally) change dosage of medication because of physical issues with changing drug levels, and 2) when medication is ended, some clients have other severe psychiatric problems that surface when the drugs are stopped.
- *Spiritual emergencies:* They are currently in or recently had a spiritual emergency. This needs to be evaluated on a case-by-case basis.
- *Paranoid:* We recommend not working with client's who have paranoid thinking. However, this is a judgment call, based on whether they feel paranoid because of the voices, or if it is due to a separate problem.
- *Current or past treatment for any psychiatric disorder:* This depends on the therapist's judgment and training.
- *Depression:* They are currently in depression, or have had a history of depression. Be sure to check for suicidal issues not brought up by the client earlier around this issue.
- *Anxiety or Obsessive-Compulsive Disorder:* Regression therapy is difficult to use with these clients, and has the possibility of making their situation temporarily worse.
- *Evaluate the content of the voices:* Do they tell the client to do 'bad things', and if so, is the client inclined to follow through? If so, this may indicate underlying behavioral problems that may be beyond what you are competent or willing to treat.

- *Any legal issues pending:* This means court dates, custody issues, or other unavoidable breaks in treatment. Clients are required to give full disclosure on this issue, and if they don't, the therapist is not required to testify as a witness in any legal proceedings involving the client's illness. This is because the therapist showed due diligence while the client has not disclosed the information asked for.
- *Tapping therapies do not work on the client:* Tapping therapies are the simplest and least painful of all therapies. If these don't work on the client, then the therapist must have training in other trauma modalities like EMDR or WHH, and the client must be informed of what to expect.
- *Minors and wards:* If the client has a legal guardian, or in any other way is not fully legally responsible for themselves, then permission is required.

The client is NOT a suitable candidate:
- *Suicidal:* Under no circumstances work with a client who is actively suicidal. If they have attempted suicide in the past or made plans to do so, the therapist needs adequate training and client support.
- *Self-mutilation (cutting, burning, etc.):* The problem is that they may accidentally harm or kill themselves during treatment.
- *Currently delusional:* This regression process is designed for clients who hear voices but can still follow directions. Clients need to be able to demonstrate insight into the nature of their condition, e.g. recognize that the 'voices' are part of their condition rather than caused by real people or 'entities'.
- *Paranoid:* if they experience paranoid delusions, they have to be able to identify those as delusional. For example, clients who might potentially include the therapist and the process into their paranoid ideation would not be acceptable candidates. Or the client feels the voices are giving them directions they have to obey would likewise not be good candidates.
- *Violence:* For the safety of the therapist, this process is not suitable for clients who have a history of violence.
- *Physical issues* (heart condition, severe lung disease like asthma with previous hospital admissions, alcohol or substance dependency, epilepsy): The client needs to be checked for life-threatening physical problems that could be triggered if severe feelings become activated.

How about doing self-help?

How about using psycho-immunological regression techniques on your own? I'll be very clear – you need to work with a trained therapist in case problems arise. Why? Well, like cutting out your own appendix, everything might go well – but if things go wrong, that training you never got won't help you. If you go into a crisis, where are you going to go for help? Most therapists won't be willing to act like a hospital emergency ward, especially involving a powerful and unfamiliar technique.

How about some of the other non-regression processes (Body Association Technique or Tribal Block Technique) in this book? At the very minimum you should work with a therapist, at least at first, while you are learning these techniques. This is for two reasons – first, you will be taught by someone who has experience and can show you how to do it correctly if you make mistakes. More importantly, if you use these techniques and get into trouble – and some people will – you've got someone who knows you, knows what you've been doing, and can jump in during a crisis situation. Trying to search for someone who can help you while you are in crisis is a bad idea – you need to have already worked with an expert who knows this material, knows you, and knows what to do in case of problems.

The 'instant expert' problem

Surprisingly, some people after getting treatment will then go home and try to treat their partners, kids, relatives, friends, or clients. Somehow, they think they can just skip years of training and practicum as a trauma therapist. This can sometimes happen because things either went really easily when they got their treatment, or their therapist was skilled enough, like a master mechanic, that he just made it look easy. Another problem can occur because most people don't believe therapy can have any risks or issues – after all, they think "we're just talking, its not surgery". However, this is not the case! You are working here with changing your internal immunological response, and this deserves your respect in the same way that a prescription drug or a surgical procedure does.

Unfortunately, the 'instant expert' problem is also endemic in the therapy profession. A lot of people have one exposure to a technique, or read a book, and then put themselves out in the public as an expert. How can you tell if you are working with a therapist who is inadequately trained, or has no training at all? First, ask them where they got their training in this technique. Secondly, a legitimate therapist will have you read and sign both an informed consent form and a liability disclaimer. If they don't, something is wrong and you should seriously consider finding a different therapist. In most countries, it is required by law for therapists to give you an informed consent form. And if possible, you should look for a trauma therapist – that specialization is quite a bit different from say counseling couples. And finally, you should look for a 'pay for results' agreement, as discussed in the last chapter.

Deceptive advertising

Another problem that happens in the therapy field (actually, in a lot of businesses) is advertising one thing but delivering something else. This happens because a person can use a well-known, popular technique name to attract clients. But instead they do whatever they want, avoiding the pesky problem of actually having to get training. For example, when someone says they use NLP and EFT, these days it means nothing because the technique names were not trademarked, and so unscrupulous therapists simply do whatever they feel like. This is in contrast to say EMDR, which has been trademarked and maintains a high level of professional standards and training.

Obviously, due to safety concerns only a therapist who is trained in these techniques should be using them. As a client and an informed consumer, you should check that they have adequate training.

Again, another much easier way to avoid this whole problem is to only work with a therapist who 'charges for results'. In other words, if the treatment did not succeed in meeting its predefined goals, there is no fee. Obviously, having a policy like this means that your therapist is pretty confident that your treatment is going to work!

Risks in doing research

I debated for a while on whether to include this topic. The reason – people who read about *research* risks confuse it with client *treatment* risks. Essentially, it is like reading about drug testing on hapless research animals but confusing it with buying a bottle of pills over the pharmacist's counter. However, I finally decided to briefly include it because of the problem that some people will immediately want to do experimentation on themselves or worse, on others, without realizing that this may be harmful. After all, they think, "this is just some kind of psychological stuff, and doing anything like that can only help me be a better person". Well, that may be true when you talk with your favorite aunt about your personal difficulties, but it is *not* true when changing the insides of your cells, with all the involuntary homeostasis reactions and parasite issues that entails.

Thus, the development of new, more effective healing techniques, peak state processes, or disease treatment involves explorations into previously undiscovered areas of the psyche and biology of consciousness. Thus, there can be hazards and problems that have never been encountered before (or if encountered, had remained unrecognized as to cause). Folks, let me put it in less formal words so you really get it. Research in subcellular psychobiology can be dangerous, it takes a lot of testing over a long time, and you can expect your staff to get injured or even killed. This is because we're working with the same underlying mechanisms that unknowingly cause regular people to get sick or go to the hospital; and these same problems can be triggered by accident in this kind of research.

On the plus side - once you're done, you can create miracles.

Research testing protocols at the Institute

To help minimize the risks associated with investigating and creating new processes and techniques, the Institute for the Study of Peak States has several layers of precautions in effect. These precautions can be divided up into three different degrees of risk depending on your involvement with the Institute - research, professional training, or clients. New material is first developed and tested in the small Institute research group, with special attention on finding any safety problems. Then the new process is tested on a larger number of highly trained Institute certified therapists, increasing the likelihood of finding any problems due to unusual situations in rare people. Given effectiveness and a lack of problems, the process is then cautiously tested on volunteer therapist trainees (or, in the case of uncommon diseases, on volunteer patients working directly with the research staff).

This testing structure can be visualized as iterations with sequential groups of volunteers (see figure 6.1). The research team is the smallest test group; once they think the process is ready, testing starts on a larger group of Institute trained therapists; and once any new problems have been solved, testing starts on the even larger client group. On average, the safety testing procedure takes 2 years after the process has been developed and considered effective and safe by the research group. Only then is the process released to private therapists (who are trained and certified by the Institute) to use with clients.

We have one other, powerful safety and effectiveness feedback system in place that is unique to the Institute. Since all of our clinics and private certified therapists all agree to only 'charge for results', the Institute gets immediate (or long term) feedback if a process does not work (or any problems arise) from the clients who want their money back. This gives clients a real incentive to contact our clinics or their private therapist if there are any problems; and hence also gives the private therapists strong financial motivation to keep us informed if their clients return.

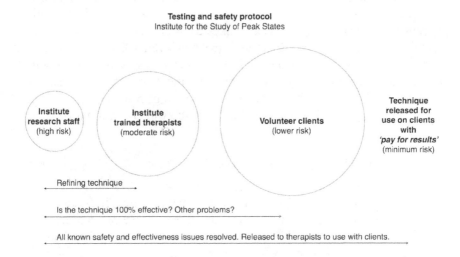

Testing and safety protocol
Institute for the Study of Peak States

Institute research staff (high risk)

Institute trained therapists (moderate risk)

Volunteer clients (lower risk)

Technique released for use on clients with *'pay for results'* (minimum risk)

Refining technique

Is the technique 100% effective? Other problems?

All known safety and effectiveness issues resolved. Released to therapists to use with clients.

Figure 6.1: A diagram of testing protocols for psychobiology techniques. From inner to outer: Research staff (very high risk); Institute trained private practice licensed therapists (moderate risk); volunteer clients (lower risk).

Risk management for Institute clinical research project volunteers

The patients who volunteer to test new clinical projects treatments for specific diseases (autism, diabetes, etc.) have their own individualized liability and risk forms depending on the condition we're working with. We use the Stanford University format for the disclosure of risk form as modified to our procedures (non-physically invasive, no drugs, etc.) The risk to the clients doing the work is relatively minimal, as we are applying (in most cases) techniques that we've worked out in other settings; and the clinic therapists are very highly trained, with advanced skills, and work directly with the research team. Empirically, after about 10 clients have been treated without any problems, we usually release the given process to the Institute clinics as a product. Usually after about 2 to 4 years of in-house experience with a process, we release it to our private practice certified therapists. If appropriate, general publication lags a few more years to give us more testing time, and because we're often too busy to take off the many months needed to write yet another book.

Safety alerts and the practitioner support forum

Over time, we occasionally find that a process that had no problems during in-house testing can have a problem for some individuals when larger groups are tested. To address this, in 2006 we established an email group so that safety announcements could be made. Over the following years, we had three safety alerts issued for processes that were taught to therapist trainees. In 2012 we switched to an online forum format for safety announcements. If you are a past or present student of the Institute, and are continuing to use the material you were taught, we highly recommend you stay signed up on the Institute's practitioner forum.

If you are a graduate of our basic Whole-Hearted Healing® therapy or PeakStates® training, we highly recommend that you sign up for our practitioner-only support discussion forum at www.PeakStates.com. It gives us a way to send out any new safety alerts, let you know about updates in technique or process changes, receive new information, ask questions or share experiences, and will help increase your professional skills. The public forum also contains current information and is searchable on the webpage.

Meet the team - Samsara Salier

Samsara writes: "I was introduced to Grant's book, *"Peak States of Consciousness"* in 2005, and very shortly after that, became the first "officially" certified graduate in The Institute for the Study of Peak States. With a background in rebirthing, this work seemed to be the next step in unravelling the secrets to good health and wellbeing."

"Because I felt my advanced skills were not as good as they could be, I decided to support the Institute by doing a lot of the behind the scenes administration work with our students and graduates around the world."

"Although the last 10 years of research has been filled with trial and error, frustration, and sometimes pain, I have hung in there, as the promise of helping to bring about a new world order has lured me on. The breakthroughs we have made along the way make it all worthwhile. We are now (hopefully... how often have we heard that?) nearing the ability to put our Humanity Project into effect. Here's hoping!"

Key Points

- All clients should read an informed consent form before starting any trauma therapy.
- Trauma therapies trigger painful emotions and sensations. Some therapies are less painful than others, although this also depends on the particular trauma experience. The fastest and least painful are meridian ('tapping') therapies.
- Some psychobiology techniques are essentially painless, but more limited in scope than trauma therapies. The body association technique is one of these.
- Eliminating all of a person's voices sometimes causes loneliness. For some people their voices, no matter how horrible, can become company for them, substituting for a lack of human connection in their lives.
- Eliminating ribosomal voices with the body association technique will also eliminate trauma induced sexual feelings. This may cause problems for intimate relationships.
- Making a person immune to the borg fungus can sometimes cause a spouse to feel like the client is no longer emotionally connected to them.
- Clients who are currently suicidal should not start treatment, as it can exacerbate their problem.
- Some people hear suicidal voices but are not in fact suicidal themselves.
- Clients using antipsychotic medications should never quit their drugs unless supervised by a physician. The drugs may be supressing other problems besides voices.
- We do not recommend these techniques for self-help.
- Potential clients should watch out for therapists without adequate training. Finding therapists who 'charge for results' is one way to find better-trained therapists.
- Research in subcellular psychobiology is potentially dangerous. Extensive testing is required before new processes are ready for use with the public.

Suggested Reading

Safety issues with prenatal regression or interacting with the primary cell:
- *Peak States of Consciousness, Volume 2* (2008) by Grant McFetridge and Wes Geitz. See appendix A for safety issues with

regression, and chapter 8 and appendix F for descriptions of prenatal developmental events.
- *Subcellular Psychobiology Diagnosis Handbook* (2014) by Grant McFetridge. See chapter 2 and 5 for parasite issues, and chapter 6 for safety issues.

Suicide issues:
- *Therapeutic and Legal Issues for Therapists Who Have Survived a Client Suicide* (2005) by Kayla Weiner ed.
- Applied Suicide Intervention Skills Training (ASIST) for suicide first aid.
- IMPACT training workshops with Dr. Iain Bourne. What makes these trainings unusually useful for suicide and mental illness is the role-playing practice they do in the courses.

Chapter 7

Other Sounds in the Mind

In this chapter, we'll cover all of the *other* (fortunately rare) mechanisms that we know of that can create voice-like phenomena. These are the 'telepathic' voices, the 'reporter' voice, and the 'one-phrase' voice. We'll follow that by discussing how subvocalization (self-talk) differs from ribosomal voices, what causes it, and how it too can be treated.

We'll also briefly mention some other phenomena that can create sounds in the mind. The most common is something we call 'sound loops' – this is experienced as playbacks of sounds, songs or voices heard over one's lifetime. Ignored by most people, this can be a severe problem for some. These playbacks are actually caused by the interactions between the mind and a parasitic ameboid organism inside the primary cell nucleus.

We'll end the chapter with a brief mention of tinnitus, and how, at least in one case it was indirectly caused by a bacterial disease that lives in the cytoplasm. We'll also mention three very rare peak abilities that have voice-like aspects – hearing the triune brains, hearing the planetary consciousness Gaia, and hearing the dead.

It is a strange and amazing world in the tiny reaches inside the primary cell.

Other voice-like diseases

As we've seen, ribosomal voices are in virtually everyone, either in their muted 'thought-like' form or in their loud, intrusive form. So this is usually the problem that clients are experiencing. However, there are a few exceptions. Over the years we've seen a small handful of other clients who had a second, totally unrelated voice-like problem. And usually their oddball voice type was their primary complaint. In the pages below we'll describe the three different types we've seen.

But before we go any further, understand that these other voice-like problems are *rare* in contrast to ribosomal voices. We've only seen a tiny handful of them. Fortunately, each type is distinctly different, so a therapist can immediately recognize them before wasting time on futile treatments. Only in one case have we had any treatment success, which surprisingly enough was by using the same body association approach we use for ribosomal voices.

Knowing that these other subcellular diseases even exist is half the battle. We hope these descriptions below spur others on to understanding the diseases involved and to create treatments.

Telepathic voices

In 2010, while I was visiting friends in California, I had the pleasure of meeting a woman who ran a support facility for mentally ill outpatient clients. Years earlier, she had suffered terribly from schizophrenic voices, and although she still had the voice problem, she was now able to function normally in life. She was remarkable, moving through her day at the facility with kindness and compassion for others who were also suffering. We chatted a bit, and she volunteered to see if I could get rid of her voices.

My techniques made no difference.

It turned out that she did *not* suffer from ribosomal voices. Instead, she experienced her voices much more like telepathy. She had a number of these telepathic presences, and unlike ribosomal voices, they would move around in space around her body, and they did not have a fixed emotional tone. Clearly, whatever was causing this problem had nothing to do with ribosomes in the ER.

Now that we knew what to look for, we have found just one other person with this same 'telepathy' problem. However, because we now rarely work with the severely mentally ill, we don't know if it is found more frequently in that group, nor if it causes more severe symptoms. These telepathic voices are not some kind of delusion – instead, we do know that they are subcellular parasites with the ability to move around inside the primary cell, but where they live and what species of disease we don't yet know.

Differential diagnosis:
Note that it is possible for people to have both the ribosomal voices and rare telepathic voices.

Telepathic voices: The client says that they are *not* like hearing people's voices, but rather are like mind reading; they move around in space; and they don't have a fixed emotional tone. This type of voice is far less common in the general population.

Ribosomal voices: By contrast, they sound like real people (who may talk, be silent, or make noises); are fixed in space; and have a fixed emotional tone. This is a very common problem.

A passionless reporter voice

Here, the person reports that they have an emotionless voice that continuously reports, like a newscaster, what is happening in their lives. I've only seen this problem three times; once in a client who had a normal life but distressed by the voice, and twice in therapists. Hence, given the number of voices clients I've seen, it is unlikely that it is a very common problem. For one person, it was quite disturbing, but for the other two it was something they were used to, albeit annoying. After testing, it was not a ribosomal voice, and honestly I have no idea what is causing it or where in the primary cell it is. (One client reported that it felt like it was speaking from the center of themselves, not from a peripheral location.)

Treatment:

We were able to treat this problem in two people. Start by eliminating all their body associations to the 'emotionless' feeling of the voice. There were several associations (in one case 5); and as each was healed, the voice's words started to drop out more and more, like a bad phone connection. Once all the associations are gone, *then* heal the generational traumas of the ancestors who also had this problem. This process fully eliminated the problem; and they reported that the change was stable when we checked back six months later.

Obviously this is *not* a well-tested treatment – if you need treatment, only work with a trained therapist who can address any unusual or unexpected problems that might arise.

Differential diagnosis:

Note that it is possible for people to have both the ribosomal voices and the passion-less reporter voice.

Passionless reporter: There is only one of these voices in a person. It has no emotional tone. It feels like it is in the center of their body. The voice is continuous, but stops when the person is about to go to sleep (as there is nothing more to report, apparently). Eliminating just one single ribosome association will not eliminate this type of voice.

Ribosomal voices: By contrast, there are usually several voices each with its own distinct emotional tone. The content of the voices ranges widely, in the same way random people in a bar might be saying different thing, nothing, or just making sounds like a grunt instead of talking. These voices don't necessarily stop even when a person is exhausted and wants to sleep.

A one-phrase swearing voice

Here is another rare, rather bizarre voice problem that we've only seen twice, once in a severely mentally ill client, the other in a therapist. The person hears a voice swearing at them with the same short phrase, for example "You're an ass!" The voice keeps saying the same thing like a trained parrot, and it can also move around inside the body. The voice has a consistent, negative emotional tone, as if someone were actually swearing at them.

We tracked the voice to a bacterium that was able to move around inside a small open area inside the nucleolus (the nucleolar vacuole). How this parasitic bacterium or bacteria is able to create a voice, and why it is like someone swearing (in the people we've seen with this problem) we don't know. Nor do we have a treatment for it yet.

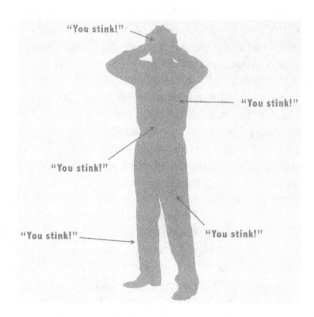

Figure 7.1: A one-phrase swearing voice.

Differential diagnosis:

Note that it is possible for people to have both the common ribosomal voices and the rare one-phrase voice.

One-phrase voice: It's verbal content is limited to only one, or sometimes two phrases. It moves around inside the body, generally in the trunk rather than in the head. It has a fixed emotional tone. There is only one voice of this type in a person.

Ribosomal voices: By contrast, they can have any verbal content that a person does, and like real people the content generally changes over time. Each voice has its own fixed emotional tone, and each voice has a fixed location in space, inside the head or outside the body or both. There are usually many voices in a person.

Subvocalization (self-talk)

When working with clients there is another issue that some people have that can be confused with ribosomal voices. We call this problem subvocalization or self-talk. In this, people are simply silently talking to themselves instead of to other people. This differs from ribosomal voices because this self-talk is exactly the same as if they were speaking aloud, except done internally to themselves. For most people, this is not a problem and they can tell the difference between the two phenomena, as this is a voluntary action that is under their control, as when rehearsing to yourself something you want to say. (A variation is when one sings or hums to themselves.) To give a feeling for the difference, imagine you are back in grade school, standing on the stage of the school auditorium. The ribosomal voices are exactly like people talking in the audience. The subvocalization is you talking on the stage. After the voices are eliminated, it is exactly like everyone has left the building and you're all alone on the stage, able to hear a pin drop. If you choose to speak, you're still in a silent, empty auditorium.

However, some people speak to themselves rather compulsively and when their ribosomal voices are gone, they still keep talking to themselves. This problem is almost always caused by straightforward, simple trauma. Essentially, the client is still trying to speak to another person with the same emotional tone that they had at the time. A slightly more indirect traumatic cause occurs if the client is subvocalizing as an attempt to suppress a feeling that they have, usually fear. (The proverbial example in the movies is a boy nervously whistling while he walks through a graveyard at night.) In this latter case, a bit more detective work might be needed to identify the relevant traumas and underlying feelings.

Example:
The client found an emotional tone of criticizing anger in the present, with a SUDS intensity of a 10. (SUDS stands for Subjective Units of Distress Scale and has a 0 to 10 range.) Regressing, he found a memory at age 45, then an earlier time, age ten. "I'm talking to someone but I don't know who it is." Using EFT, he felt energy

running in his body. Then he felt hot. "Wow, my mind is really silent, it's dead. There is nothing there, it is silent!" The therapist asked if he could get in touch with the emotional tone. "No. And I don't have the compulsion to put tension into my vocal cords, like a need to talk." Checking for other subvocalizations, he found nothing. "The subvocalization step completed the silent mind process. Before it was like going into a sound chamber, and now its like being in a silent auditorium."

In both cases the healing is still straightforward. Standard trauma techniques handle this problem, if the client wants help with this issue, or if they think that the ribosomal voices are still there because they are still compulsively self-talking. You can have the client ask themselves who in their past they might have once been talking to like this, often causing the trauma moment to pop up in their minds. Or they can simply sense the emotion driving their need to talk. In either case, a few trauma-healing experiences generally reduce or eliminate this issue adequately. Of course, one can continue this until there is no need to self-talk at all, but most clients don't bother.

Differential diagnosis:

This subvocalization problem is common in people, and can sometimes be confused with ribosomal voices.

Subvocalization: There is only one voice at a time. It feels exactly like you are talking on purpose to someone (with a slight emotional drive). It is under your control, as you can stop or start at any time, even if a feeling drives you to want to continue. The content is also your own, as you are saying to yourself what you actually feel or want.

Ribosomal voices: By contrast, the voices can have content you would not say to yourself. They also sound like other people (in the extreme, in another language), unlike your own self-talk. You can still hear them even when you have no emotional feelings of your own. They won't necessarily quit even when you are tired and want to sleep.

Sound loops: "I can't get that song out of my head"

Have you ever had a song keep running through your head that just won't stop? For many people, this happens occasionally but soon fades. However, others have a different experience. They continuously hear replays of sounds that they've heard - music, random sounds, a person's voice - and it continues on and on outside of their control. It turns out that their mind has been recording bits of what they've heard since they were a baby *in utero*, and can replay them.

To understand why this happens we need to look at the triune brains more closely. All of the triune brains in an average person act like young children in a family - and like a child with a favorite iPod, the mind brain has the ability to record and replay sounds. Usually when it replays something it is trying to be helpful, and so plays back music that it feels fit current circumstances, as if your iPod had a mind of its own. Other times it will use a recording to manipulate or dominate the rest of the triune brains, say by replaying a parent or grandparent saying a scolding word. Like ribosomal voices, for most of us these replays are muted, generally in the background and not a problem; but others suffer from this as it can be both never-ending and loud.

But it turns out that these recordings are *not* an intrinsic part of the mind. Instead, they are actually from an ameboid organism that lives inside the nucleus of the primary cell. It extrudes pseudopods out the nuclear pores; these form what looks like loops or rings on the outer surface of the nuclear membrane (see figure 7.2). These rings act very much like continuous-play eight track tapes, recording and playing back sounds that the person once heard. For most people, these 'sound loops' are clustered in one or more patches on small areas of the nuclear membrane. The mind just has the ability to tap into the content of these constantly playing sound loops at will.

Unfortunately, we don't have a treatment at this time. Around 2000 or so we developed a technique that dissolved targeted sound loops – surprisingly, after eliminating a few of the most noticeable loops thinking suddenly feels 'smooth' and not 'jangly'. Unfortunately, this technique didn't work for most people. Worse, there are a lot of sound loops, and something, either the mind brain or the ameboid organism, was not happy with us eliminating the loops. Next, we tried to heal the trauma-driven need of the mind to play these sounds back. This also failed for most clients. The third and best approach would be to make the person immune to the ameboid parasite. Unfortunately, as of this writing we've had no success yet in doing this.

Example:
The client had chronic music playing in his mind, and it never seemed to let up. Often the tone of the music was wildly different from how he was feeling, as for example when he felt afraid but was hearing a love song. Eliminating a number of the individual recordings only gave temporary relief, and after a few days the

problem returned when his emotional state stopped being as good as it had been. Eventually he found his mind brain had the feeling of wanting to escape. Using EFT on this caused a region in the back of his head to relax, and the music stopped completely.

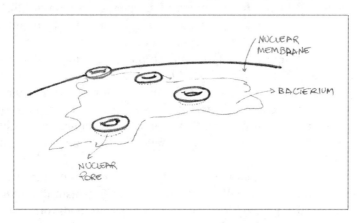

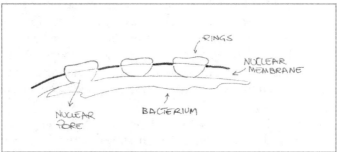

Figure 7.2: The ameboid organism (labeled as a bacteria in the illustration) that causes sound loops. Note the formation of sound loops as it extends part of its body outside the nuclear membrane through nuclear pores.

Differential diagnosis:

Note that it is possible for people to have both the common ribosomal voices and sound loops. Both are very common in people, and both are normally muted in volume.

Sound loops: They are recordings from music to voices to any sound once heard. They are relatively short, and exactly the same in each playback. There are many, many loops in the typical person. There is no emotional content other than conveyed by the tone if from someone speaking. The mind chooses which sounds to play.

Ribosomal voices: By contrast, these are sounds that could be made by real people. They seldom are repetitive, and even if so, soon change. Every voice has a fixed emotional tone. The voices say whatever they want to say, and are not controlled by the person.

Tinnitus: "A ringing in my ears"

As the Wikipedia describes it: "Tinnitus is the hearing of sound when no external sound is present. While often described as a ringing, it may also sound like a clicking, hiss or roaring. The sound may be soft or loud, low pitched or high pitched and appear to be coming from one ear or both. Most of the time, it comes on gradually. In some people, the sound causes depression, anxiety or interferes with concentration. Tinnitus is not a disease but a symptom that can result from a number of underlying causes. One of the most common causes is noise-induced hearing loss. Other causes include: ear infections, disease of the heart or blood vessels, Ménière's disease, brain tumors, emotional stress, exposure to certain medications, a previous head injury, and earwax. It is more common in those with depression. It is common, affecting about 10-15% of people. Most, however, tolerate it well, with it being a significant problem in only 1–2% of people."

We've generally had mixed success in healing this problem, probably because it may have so many different causes. In some of the clients we did help, both tinnitus and deafness led to very early trauma where the fetus heard a painfully loud noise that damaged their newly forming ear structures. (Unlike listening underwater in a bathtub, an undamaged fetus hears their mother's voice and other sounds from outside of the womb with perfect clarity.) However, at least in one case the sound was actually caused by a totally different subcellular problem, not from any ear-related damage. And some clients had negative body associations to either hearing clearly or not hearing at all that unconsciously drove them to find ways to block their hearing at the primary cell level.

Clients who come in for ribosomal voices are generally clear that tinnitus is an unrelated problem, but they should be informed that it won't be treated just in case.

Example:
A client in his 60s had very loud tinnitus in his ears. He felt the ringing sounded similar to what he'd heard after leaving loud rock concerts in his teens. Upon examination, he had a subtle sensation of what felt like earmuffs covering his ears, with a sensation that they protected his ears; the ringing came from them. These were 'copies', caused by a bacterial disease that lives in the primary cell

cytoplasm. A combination of body associations (on the earmuffs feeling) and trauma healing around the moments of copying these sounds eliminated the tinnitus. (For treating copies, see *The Whole-Hearted Healing Workbook* page 83.)

Voice-like phenomena involving peak states of consciousness

There is another class of voice-like phenomena that involve a few, uncommon states of mental health in the client – what we refer to as 'peak states of consciousness'. Out of approximately a hundred of these states, a few give people experiences that can sometimes be confused with hearing voices to an outside observer who is not trained in recognizing these phenomena. Interestingly, the people we've seen who are born with these states generally know that they are not ill, and in fact are hearing something remarkable albeit quite unusual. (Note that a person with one or more of these states is not necessarily healthy in every aspect of their lives, but for whatever reason has one or more of these unusual states of being.)

The triune brain communication peak ability

The triune brains are not only a part of us, they are self-aware in their own right. More, in very rare cases, a person can actually 'hear' their triune brains chatting with each other. Normally, a person is not conscious of this – at best, technique's like Gendlin's Focusing are used to try and communicate with the 'felt sense' of the body and heart. But there is a state of consciousness where one can actually 'hear' the brains. Although it is *not* in words, and you know this, you interpret it just as if it were spoken conversation. It can be fascinating to hear them, because one quickly realizes that they act exactly like a family of children of about age 7 or so, with boys from the sperm (right) side and girls from the egg (left) side. Because each triune brain corresponds to a different area of the body (for example, the mind brain feels like it is located in the head, the heart brain in the chest, and so on), one hears their chatter coming from these distinct locations in the physical body. And what they talk about focuses on their needs and functions, not about adult concepts (as ribosomal voices do).

More background: triune brain consciousness

The child-like quality of the triune brain consciousnesses is actually an artifact of an underlying fungal disease process in the tiny subcellular structures that house them. In extremely rare individuals these structures are immune to the disease, and so are experienced as sacred beings, as one might see or feel if one had a living totem pole extending through one's body. For more on this, we refer you to Volume 2 of *Peak States of Consciousness*.

Treatment is problematic because hearing your brains communicate is not actually a disease, but rather a very uncommon peak ability. In fact, we have a technique that gives some people the state that allows them to hear and talk with their triune brains (which is why we know this ability exists). As one might imagine, this can be a mixed blessing. It can be very useful, say as a far better substitute for dowsing, as now you're chatting directly with the body instead of using a dowsing tool to do it. But now you can't shut them off either; occasionally they're like children who want something and are having a temper tantrum. Fortunately, for the most part they simply don't have much to say.

Hearing one's triune brains is a rare situation, and so far we've only seen it in a few people, all of whom are exceptionally mentally well and extremely functional. Too, the people who can hear them somehow know that they are part of themselves. As one adult physician put it, "I've heard them since I was a little girl. They're like my family."

Differential diagnosis:

Note that it is possible for people to have both the common ribosomal voices and to hear brain communication.

Brain communication: The person knows that they are not speaking in words, even though the person comprehends them in words. Their locations correspond to places along the vertical axis of the body (from perineum to crown). They are often split left to right, with the ones on the left feeling female, the ones on the right feeling male. They seem like young children. Each focuses on what is important to their function (procreation, connection, survival, etc.). This is a very, very rare situation.

Ribosomal voices: By contrast, the voices sound like real people talking. They can be men or women, but generally not children. They are generally located in space around the head or body, not in a vertical column inside the trunk. This is a very common situation.

The Gaia communication peak ability

James Lovelock's Gaia Hypothesis, that life on earth works together to keep our planet at approximately the same average temperature is now an accepted part of climatology. Most people assume that this homeostasis is done without conscious direction. However, just as First Nations people might tell you, there *is* a planet-wide Gaia awareness, and it simultaneously interacts with everything alive on the planet, attempting to guide each organism to grow and work properly together. How do we know this is true? It turns out that there is an exceptional state of consciousness where you can actually 'hear' Gaia guiding you. We call this the 'Gaia communication' ability.

People who have this state naturally are able to 'hear' Gaia telling them what to do. Although this can be worrisome for clients who acquire this ability unexpectedly (by experimentation with hallucinogens, powerful therapies, or other causes), it is a state of health, not illness. Gaia communications are intrinsically positive, and have a unique, short syntax that is generally a command of one sort or another designed to trigger biological actions. These 'Gaia commands' do sound like they're being said in a spoken language, although bilingual people can hear them in either language. They have a distinct, unique 'echo' quality, as if a chorus were saying the words.

This ability/state isn't something that can be eliminated, nor should you want to. Educating the client so they understand what is happening is helpful. However, care must be taken to be sure that your client actually has this state, and is not just romanticizing a ribosomal or triune brain 'voice'. The three peak abilities described in this section 'sound' quite unmistakably different to someone who has experienced them – and Gaia does *not* sound like a disembodied ribosomal voice.

Differential diagnosis:

This is a *very* rare peak state of consciousness. A person can have both the state and ribosomal voices. People with voices sometimes mistakenly assume that they are hearing Gaia.

Gaia communication: The sound is unique, like a chorus from every living thing on earth speaking to you all at once from all around you. The words are short, positive, and command you to act physically or biologically to keep you healthy or in harmony with others and the world around you.

Ribosomal voices: By contrast, ribosomal voices sound just like people. They come from fixed locations in space, and there is no choral/echo effect.

Hearing the dead

Although many people report feeling the presence of departed loved ones, a few find that they can converse, in words, with the dead. This is possible because people's awareness has a physical substrate found inside the nucleus of the primary cell – as long as this material is still intact, the dead person experiences themselves as merely being 'out-of-body'. After death, the person quickly loses interest in their former life as this material substrate loses cohesion and spreads out; this dissolving process is usually finished by about a week or two after death. In rare cases, the dead person can deliberately maintain their awareness for quite some time, even up to several years, but this is by far the exception, not the norm.

The particular peak state of consciousness that allows people with it to 'verbally' communicate with the dead we call the 'God/Goddess state'. Fascinatingly, the person with this state hears the dead person speaking with exactly the same tone and voice quality that the departed had when they were living, even when they never knew what the person sounded like before death. A person with this state can talk to any dead person who is also interested in talking to them; for the most part, this means they generally only hear dead people who they knew and cared for in life in the generally short time that the dead person's consciousness can still communicate.

Since this ability is a state of health, there is no 'cure' for it. However, people with this ability may need support in dealing with the additional grief that can arise as their loved ones soon loses interest in their former life as their consciousness slowly expands and dissolves – in essence, they experience their loved one 'dying' twice. However, therapists need to remember that this ability is *rare*; people may claim they have this ability for financial reasons (as in the mediumship craze in England in the 19th century) or imagine it due to their emotional pain (loss and despair causing the person to imagine their loved one is still present).

Differential diagnosis:
Talking with the dead is a very rare ability, part of the God/Goddess peak state.

Talking with the dead: The dead person 'sounds' just like the person who has died, with their personality intact. Conversations are 'verbal' as if the dead person was still alive. The person with the ability can't just start talking to the dead person: the dead person has to choose to be in their presence, and the dead person also has to be interested in talking to them. From the perspective of the dead person, they are 'out-of-body', and usually spend their remaining time being with loved ones. For the most part, the dead relatively quickly lose interest in this life and dissolve away.

Ribosomal voices: By contrast, the ribosomal voices are like random, real people and so can pretend to be a departed person. But they are in fixed locations in space with a fixed emotional tone, and the client can 'hear' that they don't sound or feel very much like the departed person.

Tip for therapists:
The therapist can also use the simple, rapid body association technique on the voice of the 'dead person' to test if it is actually just a ribosomal voice; but both therapist and client need to be prepared for the client's reactions if their voice is eliminated.

Key Points

- There are three other, far less common, voice-like diseases that cause clients distress. They are: 'telepathic voices'; a passionless reporter voice; and a one-phrase swearing voice. These are distinctly different from ribosomal voices and can be easily identified.
- We do not yet have a treatment for the 'telepathic voices' problem. We do know it is caused by a subcellular parasite disease.
- Subvocalization (self-talk) is sometimes confused with ribosomal voices. This is quite different, and is driven by emotional trauma. Self-talk is what a person says to themselves, and is totally under their control, in the same way as their speaking voice is.
- Sound loops are playbacks of sounds heard from anytime in a person's life. They are triggered by the mind brain, but recorded in a bacterial or ameboid disease found in the nucleus. The name comes from the appearance of the structures attached to the outer surface of the nucleus.
- Tinnitus has many different possible causes. In one case, we found it was actually due to a subcellular organism that the client was unconsciously using to try and 'protect' his ears.
- There are several *rare* peak abilities that can be confused with hearing voices: triune brain communication, Gaia communication, and talking with the dead. These are states of health, not illness.
- The triune brains communicate with each other, and some rare individuals can hear them do this. However, although it is translated into words, the person knows they are not 'speaking' in words.
- People with the rare Gaia communication state 'hear' what sounds like all of the organisms in the planet telling them what to do biologically for their optimum wellbeing.
- The rare ability to talk with the dead is part of the God/Goddess state. However, people with this ability seldom realize they have it because it generally manifests only with their newly departed friends and loved ones.

Summary Table of 'Other Sounds in the Mind'

	Type	Cause	Treatment	Prevalence
Ribosomal voices (pp. 69)	'Audible' voices	Borg fungus via ribosomes.	Body associations or Silent Mind Technique.	Almost all humans.
Telepathic voices (pg. 104)	Not 'audible' voices	Unknown – we suspect a prion disease origin.	None known at this time.	Rare.
Reporter voice (pg. 105)	'Audible' voice	Unknown – probably fungal.	Body associations and generational healing	Very rare.
One-phrase swearing voice (pg. 106)	'Audible' voice	Unknown.	None known at this time.	Rare.
Subvocalization (pg. 107)	Self-talk speaking voice	Biographical trauma	Biographical trauma healing.	Very common; seldom an issue.
Sound loops (pg. 108)	Speech fragments and other sounds	Ameboid organism in nucleus.	None known at this time.	Very common; seldom an issue.
Tinnitus (pg. 111)	Various non-voice sounds	Many different causes.	No single treatment (see text).	Relatively common; seldom an issue.
Triune brain communication (pg. 112)	Interpret as voice-like	A peak state – can hear triune brains.	Is a state of health. Possible adjustment issues.	Very rare.
Gaia communication (pg. 113)	Interpret as voice-like chorus	A peak state – can hear Gaia commands.	Is a state of health. Possible adjustment issues.	Very rare – usually felt as 'intuition'.
Hearing the dead (pg. 114)	'Audible' voice	A peak state - can hear the dead speak.	Is a state of health. Possible adjustment issues.	Very rare.

Suggested Reading

For more on peak abilities and peak states of consciousness:

- *Peak States of Consciousness*, Volume 2 (2008) by Grant McFetridge and Wes Gietz.

For more on subcellular parasitical organisms that affect the psyche:

- *Subcellular Psychobiology Diagnosis Handbook* (2014) by Grant McFetridge. See chapter 2 for an overview of subcellular parasite diseases.

For detailed diagnostic criteria for therapists (including ICD-10 categories):

- *Subcellular Psychobiology Diagnosis Handbook* (2014) by Grant McFetridge. See chapters 8-13 and appendix 11 for detailed descriptions of various subcellular diseases and their diagnosis.

Chapter 8

New Horizons

Because I wanted a simpler and better way to make people immune to the borg fungus, I put off writing this book for several years even after I developed the fast and simple body association technique (described in Chapter 5). In 2017 I finally decided to write this book anyway, as our existing techniques would still help many people. Only weeks into the book, my team and I came up with a prototype technique that looks like it will be a better, simpler, and more effective way to get rid of the fungus. It will take a year or two before we've thoroughly tested it, but so far, it looks like what I was hoping to find.

In this chapter I'm going to give you a peek into this ongoing research process.

The need for a better borg fungal immunity process

Our current regression technique (revision 2.3) to make people immune to the borg fungus is pretty reliable at this point, but it has some serious drawbacks. First, it isn't easy – it needs a trained therapist to work with the client. Secondly, it involves experiencing pain and suffering. Third, it really doesn't address the other symptoms of mental illness, albeit it is useful for typical people who want a silent mind or want to get rid of the tribal block problem. Forth, it does not always work (the failure rate is a bit hard to be sure of, but it looks to be roughly 5% in our relatively healthy client population). Over the next few years I tried various new approaches, but none of them worked better than the revision 2.3 regression approach.

This last problem, that some people did not get the silent mind result after using the technique, had me very concerned because I didn't know why this was happening. When I looked into it, I found that some clients would report that their mind was not silent because they were experiencing unrelated problems (see chapter 7 for more on this). However, our technique really did not work for some people. I also knew there was still a theoretical gap in my model. The technique was working at a moment in development when the borg fungus was already present. When, exactly did a person first get infected, and why? If I could find that moment, I might be able to make a better technique.

Tracking the borg fungus to the first infection

It was in early 2015 I was finally able to answer these questions. I had the good fortune to work with two exceptional men who'd taken training from the Institute. Both were unable to get the silent mind state, they understood what I was trying to do, and they were willing to experiment. So we met for buffet breakfasts over several days at the wonderful Kolanko's restaurant in Krakow, Poland, and while eating and chatting we'd work together on this problem. And we got lucky. One of them had a walled off area in the pre-organelle cell that was still loaded with fungus. The technique had cleared the rest of the cell, but the person would stay infected because the fungus would still be released later.

But with the other fellow we hit pay dirt. His problem was quite different. He had a giant fungal organism almost filling the pre-organelle cell, and just couldn't dissolve it fully. To give a feeling for scale, imagine the first fellow had a swimming pool with a bunch of leaves in one corner, while the second had a pool with an entire whale in it. Up to now, when we'd regressed to try and find the originating problem, we'd get lost in all the possible places it seemed to be from, as these fungal organisms were quite tiny and all over the place in those earlier events, like leaves in a windy fall day. However, this whale-sized fungus was a lot easier to track to its origin.

To explain where this took us, I'll need to review some subcellular biology we'd worked out using regression and observations of the primary cell. At the center of the person's nucleus is a structure that looks somewhat like a First Nations totem pole. This tiny structure is made up of 14 roughly cubical block-like structures, each one controlling a subcellular organelle and its corresponding body system and brain structure. Seven of these blocks come from the father, seven from the mother. These blocks bud from the parental blocks when the parent is still a newly implanted zygote starting to make primordial germ cells (that later become sperm or eggs).

As we tracked that fellow's giant fungus further into the past, it took us to his newly budded body block. It was damaged in what felt like his navel area – a hole was left where it had separated from its parental block. As this new block first moved away from its parental block, a free-floating borg fungal organism was abruptly pulled into the hole, as if jamming a cork into a wine bottle. This observation explained a lot; the body felt it needed the fungus for what felt like its survival, and so wasn't about to get rid of it. This also explained why a person in the present had the tribal block effect in what feels like their navel.

A failed attempt

My immediate reaction was to find ways to seal up the body block's hole to keep the borg fungus out. However, there were several huge potential problems with trying to close this hole. The first is the risk of suicide. Because the block hole feels like it is at the navel of the regressed person, we were concerned that a process that focused on it might unintentionally trigger umbilical cord-cutting trauma. Decades ago we'd found that a person could suddenly become suicidal if they consciously or unconsciously accessed the cord-cutting experience – even if they'd never felt suicidal before. Worse, this trauma can sometimes express as a calm, emotionless drive for suicide that does not give any warning signs (the person unknowingly identifies with the placenta's need to die during the birth process). It is no exaggeration to say that working with a problem like this is like wearing a blindfold and strolling through a field of land mines. The second problem is potentially just as bad – this very early event involves several very dangerous parasitic species that can also negatively influence a person's psyche and health. Working in this time zone can trigger severe problems in the present due to new parasite interactions and parasite overgrowth.

Very cautiously, I came up with a way to close the hole to get rid of the borg fungus, but in our volunteers the hole would stay closed for only a short time, on the order of minutes to days. Then it would open again and the borg problem would be back. However, this testing did show us something very important and unexpected. If someone does close their navel hole, they would instantly and continuously feel safe and loved. I tested this on about a dozen volunteers with the same result. Aha, I thought, this might really make a difference for people with mental illness!

Cautious optimism

As of this writing two years later, we now feel we understand how and why the navel hole exists, and are working on a new prototype treatment. But one never knows how long it will take to develop (or if it will work at all) when doing research into new territory. And of course, once we've got something that works on our research staff, we're going to have to do a lot of very cautious testing to make sure it does not evoke suicidal feelings in some people. On the positive side, there is a good chance that the new technique will be much easier and hopefully much safer to do. Eliminating this navel hole problem will likely also eradicate a number of other less common disorders and subcellular diseases. Cross your fingers that this works out like we hope!

This new borg fungus immunity process development is actually just a side project for us. Instead, much of our time is spent on finding a way to eliminate *all* fungal diseases simultaneously. Assuming we're successful, it will be interesting to see how these two different approaches play out in the future.

Meet the team - Shayne McKenzie, our CEO

Shayne writes: "For as long as I can remember, I have been interested in optimal health - not just physical health but health in all areas of life. During my career, this interest has led me to study many different areas, undertake numerous personal development courses, and be trained and certified in a number of leadership tools and several alternative therapies."

"It was about 10 years ago that I went to an information session on Peak States of Consciousness. I immediately felt like this was the information that I was looking for that would explain the different psychological states that people experienced. I signed up for the next training session in 2008 and after a very comprehensive training and assessment process became a certified therapist in 2009."

"Since then I have seen my clients have extraordinary results with Peak States therapy. The issues that have been addressed have ranged from permanently eliminating the emotional pain associated with years of depression to a decade of chronic back pain disappearing after only three sessions. I have also helped many people attain extraordinary peak states, which has helped them experience a much more positive and healthy life. This work that I was now doing truly felt meaningful. I particularly like that this approach addresses the underlying biological cause rather than just the symptoms - a key thing I was looking for in my journey to understand optimal health. I was also moved and inspired when I heard about many more examples from other Peak States therapists achieving similar results."

Meet the team – Shayne McKenzie (continued)

"Given the significant difference that this was making to humanity, I wanted to do more than just help my clients. I wanted to use my business and people leadership skills in a way that would make the most meaningful impact on humanity. I wanted to help spread the word of this breakthrough biological model and the very effective treatments that could make such an impact on people's lives. Therefore, last year, I took on the role of CEO for the Institute for the Study of Peak States. My key goal is to increase the awareness of Peak States therapy so that many more people can experience optimal health. This is a life that inspires me and is driven by a meaningful purpose. I hope that our vision of making such a fundamental positive impact on humanity is realized in my lifetime."

Key Points

- The current revision 2.3 regression technique for eliminating the borg fungal infection has several drawbacks, and doesn't work for everyone (roughly 5% of the healthy client population tested did not become immune; we assume a higher failure rate will occur with mentally ill client populations).
- The borg fungus is acquired in the parental primary cell at the very beginning of the creation of primordial germ cells.
- The borg fungus is present in most people because the body mistakenly believes it needs it for its survival.
- Research in early developmental events is potentially dangerous due to subcellular parasite interactions or other unintended consequences.
- Umbilical cord-cutting trauma can trigger suicide feelings or actions in many people.

Suggested Reading

About risks with research in subcellular psychobiology:
- "Going public with subcellular psychobiology" (2014), by Dr. Grant McFetridge. This is a blog post at Peak States.com, about the

problems we had to solve before we felt this information was safe to present to the public.

About the medical implications of subcellular psychobiology:

- "Epigenetics, psychoneuroimmunology, and subcellular psychobiology" (2016) by Dr. Grant McFetridge. This is a blog post at Peak States.com, about psychobiology techniques that interact with subcellular phenomena.
- "Snake oil, or the real deal?" (2016) by Dr. Grant McFetridge. This is a blog post at Peak States.com, talking about this new field of subcellular psychobiology.
- "Subcellular psychobiology is a 'disruptive technology'" (2016) by Dr. Grant McFetridge. This is a blog post at Peak States.com, about how disruptive technologies work.
- "Where are the 'medical' applications?" (2016) by Dr. Grant McFetridge. This is a blog post at Peak States.com, about the confusion some have around mental disorders without an obvious causal disease.

About the subcellular block structures and their pre-organelles:

- *Peak States of Consciousness, Volume 1* (2004) by Grant McFetridge et al. See chapters 5 and 6.
- *Peak States of Consciousness, Volume 2* (2008) by Grant McFetridge and Wes Geitz. See chapters 3 and 11.

Section 3

Appendices

Appendix A

A 'Pay for Results' contract

Predetermined criteria contract for the Silent Mind Technique

The Silent Mind Technique is a process that therapists use with clients to eliminate all ribosomal voices. For this process the Institute specifies predetermined criteria, although the therapist can adjust the document as needed to fit the client's wording and situation. Of course, the therapist needs to evaluate the client before treatment starts to be sure their problem is due to ribosomal voices.

If the therapist instead uses only the Body Association Technique for elimination of just one or a few voices, this agreement will need to be appropriately modified. Likewise, if only the Tribal Block or Distant Personality Release techniques are used, the therapist would also change the agreement.

For an in-depth description of how to use the 'pay for result' way of working with psychotherapy clients, see chapter 3 and Appendices 2 and 10 in our *Subcellular Psychobiology Diagnosis Handbook*.

***

Dear --------,

Thank you for signing the liability and informed consent forms, and filling out your patient history form.

We're scheduled to work with you at your 6pm (*appointment time*). As we discussed, we'll need to do the treatment three times - the first time should get rid of your voices, but by the next day they may return. We do a second treatment 2 to 4 days later, and then a final check (and minor treatment if needed) in about 2 weeks to make sure the problem does not return.

This is a 'pay for results' agreement - this means if we don't meet our agreement, there is no fee. Note that we do not agree to eliminate other issues. As we also discussed, we do not know if your visual hallucinations will be eliminated or not. You should expect that they will not go away with this treatment.

AGREEMENT

We agree to eliminate the client's intrusive voice chatter; i.e., background thoughts you hear when you are trying to meditate (that can sound like other people's voices). We will test the results by having the client meditate for a few minutes and listen. These voices feel like they are in fixed locations in space, and have fixed emotional tones.

After the process, the client will have the sensation that their head feels empty, quiet, open and large (like they are now standing on an empty stage). Note that you will soon become used to this feeling and it will be hard to notice it later.

The fee is $------- payable in 3 weeks after the change is stable. If the voices return, and a follow-up treatment does not work, there is no fee.

Post Treatment Care

If treatment is successful, you might have a reaction to losing your voices. Although infrequent, some clients have feelings of loneliness after their voices leave. If you have this issue, please let us know so we can treat it in the follow-up sessions. Some find that people they are close to (spouses in particular) feel like you are now more distant or aloof, even though you have not changed. This is a normal outcome, due to the fact you don't unconsciously connect to them in the same way. This issue passes with time as they adjust to your new condition. In some cases, your sexual attraction to your spouse may be reduced or lost – this also generally comes back over time as you both adjust to the changes.

If you are taking medication, you must work with your physician to determine if you should change dosages. Do not stop any medication abruptly without the advise of your health care provider. Stopping some medications quickly is dangerous and can cause severe symptoms. Remember, even though your voices may now be gone, your medication may have also been treating some other problem that could still be present.

If you have any other problems arise as an immediate outcome of treatment, contact us immediately. My phone is ------------.

Sincerely,
Signed -----------

Date:

Client Signature:

Appendix B

Frequently Asked Questions

Q: What is the 'Silent Mind Technique'?
A: That is what we call our voices elimination process. Depending on the client's situation, we use several different techniques developed for this purpose.

Q: How long does the Silent Mind Technique take? How many treatment sessions?
A: The treatment is usually finished in one or two office visits; then we have two short follow-up visits to be sure we healed the problem fully. Treatment time can range from a minimum of about an hour, to a maximum of about 9 hours.

Q: What technique do you use for the treatment?
A: Psychological techniques that heal post-traumatic stress disorder (PTSD) symptoms that occurred in pre-natal development.

Q: Is medication used in the treatment?
A: No. We only use Peak States therapy techniques.

Q: Does the treatment have to be repeated regularly?
A: No. The results are permanent – the treatment does not have to be repeated.

Q: Will follow up treatments be required?
A: No, after the first sequence of treatments, the result is permanent.

Q: If my mind is silent, can I still think?
A: Yes. You can still deliberately subvocalize to yourself to rehearse what you want to say to someone; or still recall catchy tunes.

Q: Does the treatment hurt?
A: Depending on the technique used, there can be some brief emotional and physical pain as injuries that were acquired prenatally are re-experienced and eliminated.

Q: How will I feel between sessions?
A: It is very individual how the clients feel between treatments. Most are free of symptoms after the first appointment; others need the second treatment.

Q: What do you mean by saying you 'charge for results'?
A: Just like it sounds - if the treatment doesn't work, there is no charge to you.

Q: Will I miss my voices?
A: Even though the voices were a torment for many people, some miss them after they are gone. Fortunately, this distressing feeling can also be eliminated, leaving the client feeling peaceful that the voices are gone.

Q: Can I expect to be healed, or does the treatment only help some people?
A: In our testing so far, our treatment works on most people. However, there are also other, much less common voice-like disorders – your therapist will check to see if you have them before starting treatment.

Q: Can I quit taking my drugs immediately after treatment?
A: No. You need to work with your physician with regards to changing your drug treatment. For example, many people experience severe withdrawal symptoms if they abruptly end drug treatment; or your drug treatment may be helping you handle a different psychological problem.

Q: Are there any side effects to the treatment?
A: Possibly. If the treatment is successful, some clients may have usually minor adjustment issues afterwards. These include loneliness because the voices are gone, upset partners because you may suddenly feel distant to them, and sounds becoming louder and more distinct.

Q: Why haven't I heard about this treatment from my doctor?
A: The process is still very new, and not many people know of these techniques yet. We expect that it will take years for this new breakthrough to become common knowledge.

Q: If I have more questions, where can I get an answer?
A: You are welcome to phone or e-mail the Institute.

Q: Does the Silent Mind Technique cure all schizophrenics?
A: No. The treatment only addresses *one* of the key symptoms of schizophrenia (that of ribosomal voices) that many schizophrenics have. It generally does not eliminate other non-voice symptoms (although occasionally it will because their other symptoms were indirectly caused by the presence of the voices).

Appendix C

Informed Consent Form

Therapist's Name:
Mailing Address:
Office Phone:
Office Email:
Office Hours:

Hello,

We're going to start our work together by going over this informed consent form. Many countries have laws requiring that we do this; but it is a good idea to do anyway, as it may answer some of your questions, or address ones you may not have even thought about before. As we cover each item, I'll have you check it off to show that you and I discussed it to your satisfaction. I'll keep the original form, and give you a copy for your records.

What are my qualifications and orientation as a therapist?

When you need your car engine fixed, you need to go to a mechanic who knows all about engines – you don't go to the transmission guy. In the same way, therapists also specialize, and are better at some things than others; and some things they just don't have the right training for. Thus, I am what is known as a trauma therapist, specializing in healing traumatic memories that you may or may not realize cause you problems. Later, during our discussion of 'pay for results', we'll go over your issue to see if I feel I can help you with your particular problem; but for now, here's a description of my formal background:

- Academic qualifications:

    _____.

- My formal certification as a therapist or counselor is by (in)
  _____.
- I am certified by _____ to
  use their techniques.
- Professional membership(s):
  _____.
- Therapeutic orientations:
  _____.

❏ We've discussed what my therapist's qualifications and therapeutic orientation, and I understand what the therapist is saying.

What issues won't I work with?

There are certain issues that I will be sending you to see another therapist for. The most important for you to know about is the issue of suicide. If you have suicidal feelings, have attempted to commit suicide, or have made plans to commit suicide, you need to see someone else who specializes in this problem. If this comes up during our work together, I will end our sessions and refer you to another therapist (or other professional) who works with this issue.

   Another problem that might come up involves physical problems like heart conditions. Because therapy might bring up strong emotional and physical reactions, if you have any medical conditions that might put you at risk, we cannot start therapy.

❏ We've discussed the areas that my therapist won't work with, and I understand and agree to this. Additionally, I don't have any of the suicidal issues that we discussed, nor do I have any physical condition (like heart troubles) that might be triggered by therapy.

Confidentiality and its exceptions

During our sessions, I may be taking written notes, or audio or video recordings. This helps me remember what we accomplished or still need to do; and can help remind you too, because one of the common effects of modern therapy is forgetting what one's issue used to be (the 'apex effect'). This material is confidential and is not for other people, even after we finish working together. However, there are some exceptions:

   a) If a child is or may be at risk of abuse or neglect, or in need of protection;

b) If I believe that you or another person is at clear risk of imminent harm;

c) For the purpose of complying with a legal order such as a subpoena, or if the disclosure is otherwise required or authorized by law.

d) If you are in couples therapy with me, do not tell me anything you wish kept secret from your partner.

e) I may also disclose information for the purpose of a professional consultation, or for a professional presentation or paper, in which case your identity will remain confidential. *(Note: if you are a client at an Institute clinic, your full information is available to other Institute staff as needed.)*

f) I may also be sharing anonymous data (length of time, effectiveness, unusual problems) from our sessions to help improve the quality of the processes we are using.

g) You should be aware that email or cell phones can be monitored by others, so don't communicate in this way if you wish confidentiality.

❑ We've discussed exceptions to confidentiality, and I understand and agree with these terms of therapy.

Benefits and risks of trauma therapy

The trauma-based therapy that we will be doing is intended to heal the specific issue(s) that you and I decide on in our 'pay for results' agreement. Trauma therapy may also bring deeper personal insight and awareness, solutions to, or better ways of understanding and coping with problems, improved relationships, significant reductions in feelings of distress, and greater insight into personal goals and values.

You should know, however, that trauma therapy usually requires that you be willing to examine and discuss difficult topics or times in your life, to experience stronger than usual emotions, and to try out new and different behaviors. The therapy may feel challenging and difficult at times. Uncomfortable feelings and experiences may be addressed (in that you may feel anger, sadness, guilt, grief, loss, frustration, etc.) as well as physical discomforts or pains (nausea, aches, pains). During treatment, you may feel worse before you start to feel better. And I simply may not be able to help you, or, in rare cases, the therapy may make you feel worse than when we started. However, you ultimately get to decide what we discuss and work with. If you feel uncomfortable or not ready to discuss a particular issue at any point, this is completely okay.

In your session, we'll almost certainly be using one or more state-of-the-art therapies such as EMDR, EFT, TAT, TIR, or WHH, depending on your issue and other factors. (They work far better than older trauma techniques.) You should also know that these techniques, although widely used, are still considered experimental and may cause you problems that have not yet been recognized. Also, the techniques you might learn in therapy are for your own use and not to be taught to others, be they partners, family, friends, therapists or clients. This is for their safety, because formal training is needed in case something goes wrong; and also because some of these techniques are trademarked.

There are other different types of therapy you might want to pursue instead. For example, you might simply need a counselor to help you come to a decision in your life, and not someone to heal the feelings you have around the situation. If you decide to continue, we'll look at the issue you want to heal, and decide if it is something we can agree on treating, and ways to measure success. And of course, after this discussion, you may realize that not doing anything is the right thing for you at this time.

❑ We've discussed therapy's benefits, risks, and other options available to me, and I understand and choose to continue with trauma therapy.

Benefits and risks of Peak States processes

There is another kind of therapy, where the focus is on gaining certain 'peak states' of consciousness. For example, you can get a continuously quiet mind, or a feeling of peace that is greater than normal.

So, what are the difficulties or risks with using these processes? First, they involve healing prenatal trauma. If you don't heal them fully, you may feel badly for a period of time ranging from hours to days, and perhaps longer, until these memories re-submerge and leave your awareness. Secondly, these processes are relatively new and experimental. Long-term effects, if any, have not been studied or researched. This means that there is always the possibility that problems may occur that we have never seen before, and do not know how to deal with. By analogy, this is like a new drug that after a few years turns out to have side effects that only affected some people. If problems happen, I will call in specialists to help, but even they may not be able to solve your problem. Given this, why would you ever want to use such a process? The reason is the same as why you would use a new drug – it can do things that you really want done, and there are no obvious problems (at least so far).

Obviously, due to safety concerns only a therapist who is trained in these techniques should be using them. If you go ahead with this type of treatment, you must not share the techniques with others, including your spouse or other therapists you know.

❑ We've discussed the Peak States processes benefits and risks. I understand that there may be problems that remain after the treatment is finished. [Circle the choice that applies to you below:]
- • Yes, I am willing to accept the risks and any consequences that may arise, and use these processes. I agree not to share the techniques with anyone else (including friends and family).
- • No, I am unwilling to accept the risks or be fully responsible for what happens, and so will not use the processes.

Practical details

If you decide to start therapy, we will start by writing up a 'pay for results' agreement for your therapy. Sessions are typically two hours long, but can run overtime; and we'll agree on a schedule that works for both of us. If you miss three sessions without canceling or with less than 24 hour notice, or cancel therapy before completion (up to five sessions), you may forfeit your deposit (if any). I do not do insurance billing.

I encourage you to phone if any emergency situations arise from our work between sessions, but other concerns should be addressed in your regular therapy session. My phone number is at the end of this document. When I am unavailable or on vacation, I will provide you with a contact number of someone who can assist you.

If you have a life-threatening emergency, you must either call the Suicide and Crisis Hotline at _____, phone emergency services at ___911 in the US and Canada___, or go to the nearest emergency room. I provide only non-emergency therapeutic services by scheduled appointments. If I may need additional or more intensive services, I may refer you to another organization to receive extended services.

❑ We've discussed practical details of our work together, especially about emergencies, and I understand and agree to these terms.

Reviews, referrals and ending

In counseling, it is your right at any time to:
- a) Have a review of your progress and of any of the topics in this form;
- b) Be provided with a referral to another counselor or health professional;

c) Withdraw consent for the collection, use, or disclosure of your personal information, except where precluded by law;

d) End the counseling or therapeutic relationship by so advising the therapist or counselor. (This may forfeit part or all of your deposit, but the amount will be less than or equal to the standard $100/hr rate of the time you've already spent in therapy.)

e) Access or obtain a copy of the information in your counseling records, subject to legal requirements.

Your right of access to or to obtain a copy of your personal information continues after the end of the counseling relationship.

I reserve the right to terminate therapy at any time. This may occur, for example, if I believe that I simply can't help you. If this happens, there would be no charge to you for our work up to that point and your deposit (if any) would be returned.

❑ We've discussed my rights around the termination of therapy, and I understand and agree to these terms.

Concerns or complaints

If you have a concern about any aspect of your counseling, I would prefer that you first address it with me. If you feel that this is impossible or unsafe, or if your concern is not resolved through our discussion, you should contact the Institute for the Study of Peak States at +1-250-413-3211. If this doesn't resolve your complaint, you should then contact the local governmental body that regulates therapists in your country.

❑ We've discussed how to deal with any complaints or problems I have with my therapist, and I understand and agree to these terms.

Signature

"My signature below confirms that I (the client) have read the above, had an opportunity to discuss it with the therapist, had sufficient time to consider it carefully, and had my questions answered to my satisfaction."

Name of Client	Name of Therapist
Signature of Client	Signature of Therapist
Date signed	Signature of Witness if any

Revisions:
2.1 April 17, 2010

Appendix D

The Body Association Technique™

Body associations are trauma-caused, illogical connections between unrelated feelings and sensations, as when Pavlov's dog salivates at the sound of a bell. The Body Association Technique (below) is used to rapidly and easily eliminate them. Although the technique can be used for a number of psychological problems, in this book we only focus on how to use it for the elimination of ribosomal voices.

Eliminating Ribosomal Voices
When using the Body Association Technique to eliminate 'voices':
- The technique dissolves one ribosomal voice at a time.
- The process is ideal for eliminating a few problem voices, as it is painless, fast, with no side effects other than potential adjustment issues to the changes (as described below).
- It can also be used to eliminate the ribosomes that cause trauma-driven sexual attractions (as these are the same ribosomes that can contain voices).
- With patience and repetition it can be used to eliminate all voices.
- This technique should be used with a therapist, but after some initial supervision it can be used for self-help. (See Chapter 6 for more details).

(Note that for a simultaneous and permanent elimination of all ribosomal voices, we currently use a regression process that is part of the Silent Mind Technique, revision 2.2. However, this process is slower, harder to do, and has more potential side effects and adjustment issues than the body association technique approach described below.)

How to eliminate a problem 'voice'
The technique has to be used in a very specific way to eliminate a ribosomal voice. In step 1 (below), have the client focus on the target 'voice' and get its emotional tone. We also recommend they identify where

in space the voice is, so that they can notice when the target voice is eliminated and not confuse it with other voices located elsewhere.

In step 2, have them find the hand that has an imaginary bag that radiates that *exact* emotion. In this case, there will only be one ribosome that will be an exact match – you do not have to repeat the process for that voice again. (Thus step 4 can be skipped, assuming they got an exact match of the voice's emotional tone with the ribosome in their hand.)

In step 3, use the Body Association Technique to do the healing. That voice will vanish from the place it was located in space, leaving the sensation of a blank or empty area there.

Healing a sexual attraction to eliminate a voice

The Body Association Technique can also be used to eliminate voices in an indirect way. When a dysfunctional sexual attraction is eliminated, a corresponding ribosomal voice will also be eliminated. Not every attraction has a voice associated with it, but they all can potentially become voices in the future. Thus, eliminating them all is a good proactive step. Too, these powerful, dysfunctional attractions cause havoc in people's lives, so eliminating them is a very good idea.

For step 1, have the client focus on anyone they have a *sexual* attraction towards. This can be people they know, or actors from movies. Have the client notice the other person's most dominant emotional tone (angry, sad, happy, etc.). Ignore the client's response to the other person's emotional tone. For example, the other person may feel angry to the client, which makes the client feel defensive or rejected. The correct feeling to use in the technique would be the *other* person's anger, not the client's feeling.

Use steps 2 and 3 on this emotion until the association is healed. The client will suddenly no longer feel any physical sexual attraction to them if you eliminated the correct emotional association. There is only one ribosome per sexual attraction. If there is still some sexual attraction left, repeat the process (step 4) to eliminate the correct emotional tone.

Since these attractions are irrationally associated with survival, we suggest picking the strongest attractions first, as they probably cause the most problems in the client's life.

Potential adjustment issues with eliminating ribosomal voices:

In our experience there are no side effects from the Body Association Technique itself. However, there might be adjustment issues *after* eliminating voices.

- For example, if you accidentally heal the associations you have to your partner's emotional tones, you may temporarily loose your sexual attraction to your partner. Clearly, if this emotional addiction was the only reason you are with your partner, you may be facing major adjustment issues.

- Another potential problem is sudden feelings of loneliness appearing with the abrupt absence of the voice(s). The therapist should check at the end of the process to see if this has arisen – if so, use standard techniques (such as EFT) to eliminate this feeling of loneliness.

If you eliminate *all* of your ribosomal voices with this approach, some people may have the following potential issues appear. (See Chapter 6 for an in-depth discussion.)

- Sounds and voices suddenly seem louder, sometimes a lot louder.
- A voice may be missed because it was silent when you were focusing on them.
- A new voice may suddenly appear later. You will notice either thoughts appearing or the feeling of sudden heaviness if you are suppressing it.

Body Association Technique™
Revision 2.0, Feb 22, 2013

Step 1: Identify the potential target sensation or emotion
Have the client identify the sensation or emotion that may have an association.

In this technique, it is not necessary to find what the other associated feelings are. Instead, if you suspect that there is an association, you can simply target the sensation that the client can feel – all other associated feelings will be eliminated automatically by the technique.

Associations can be anything to anything without any logical sense. And a given stuck body brain gene can cause more than a single pair of associations; for example the sensation of cold is linked to fear which is linked to the color red which is linked to... and so on. (As a simple approximation, you might think of these body associations as addictions, although they also cause many other problems.)

Examples:
Associations generally don't make any logical sense or have any pattern (except in some developmental events where the sensations are the same for everyone and so can be predicted). Thus, we've seen in clients a variety of associational problems, for example: the sensation of 'love' was associated with 'pain'; 'getting peak states' was associated with 'I'm going to die, or be annihilated'; 'trust' was

associated with 'annihilation', 'death', 'betrayal', and 'loss of control'; 'public speaking' was associated with 'I'm going to die'.

Body associations can also cause more indirect problems. For example, one client had the sensation of peace and calmness associated with death, so to avoid death this client was constantly stimulating new traumatic feelings into their awareness – causing unending drama in their life.

Step 2: Find the body association

Have the client hold out one of their hands, with the palm upwards and the fingers slightly cupped. Have them imagine that there is a 'crumpled bag' (like an empty snack bag) held in their hand. Then, have them see if they can feel that the bag radiates the target body sensation. The client will try to obey the instructions you give, but if there is not a body association, the exercise will lack any sense of reality. However, if they do have a real association, the client will find that they can actually sense that the invisible crumpled bag in their hand is radiating the sensation (or emotion) that you've targeted. This sensation is quite distinct, and once a client has experienced it, they won't be fooled by their imagination or made up experiences.

This trick with the hand simulates the sensation of the endoplasmic reticulum's pore that holds the ribosome that radiates the sensation of the association.

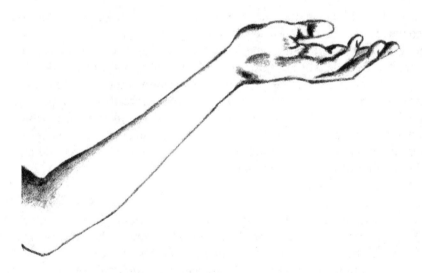

Figure D.1: Have the client hold out their hand with the fingers upright in a cupped position, as if ready to start holding something.

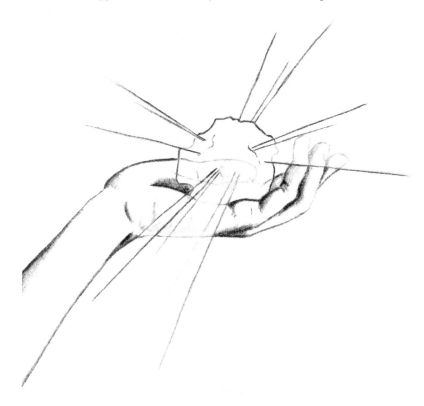

Figure D.2: Have the client sense for something like an invisible crumpled bag in their hand, that radiates the target sensation. Have them alternately check both hands to find the 'bag' that feels the most present in their imagination.

Step 3: Eliminate the body association

Have the client tap on the 9-gamut point on the back of the hand containing the imaginary crumpled bag that radiates the target sensation. The client can usually do the tapping; having the therapist do this is usually unnecessary. The typical time to dissolve an association is around 90 seconds. If it takes more than 2 minutes, stop the process because something is wrong - usually that there is no real association in that hand, and the client was just imagining one. Fortunately, we haven't seen a client yet who cannot do this process – this technique is very, very robust.

When the stuck gene releases, the 'crumpled bag' (the ribosome) will rise out of their hand and dissolve. This is usually quite a surprise to the client, because it is outside of their control – up to that point, they may have been thinking that this was just a psychological exercise in imagination. It is also a very good finish point that the therapist should be waiting for. Have the client tap fifteen more seconds or so after the bag has vanished (to more fully heal any still-damaged histone protein on the stuck gene.)

In some cases, the 'crumpled bag' only partly disappears, leaving some of the sensations that were in the bag. This was due to the problem of 'multiple roots' – more than one gene was involved with the association. (Visually, part of the ribosome dissolved, but not all of it.) In this case, simply continue tapping until the rest of the 'bag' fully vanishes.

(Instead of tapping, one can send a feeling of love and joy into one's body along the arm to do the healing. However, many clients cannot make this approach work, so we recommend the tapping instead, which works for everyone.)

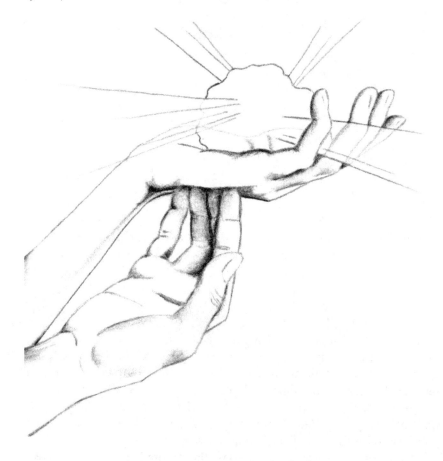

Figure D.3: Have them tap on the 9-gamut point while staying focused on the radiating feeling in the imaginary bag. (The 9 gamut meridian point is on the back of the hand between the ring finger and pinkie tendons.)

Step 4: Look for more associations

Return to the original problem. Have the client check for the same target sensation or emotion in an invisible bag in the *other* hand. (This occurs when a maternal side gene and the paternal side gene have the same association. Heal as in step 3. Then switch back to the original hand and look for another bag (ribosome) that also has the same original feeling. Heal as in step 3. Then again switch hands, continuing this pattern of healing. When you can no longer find a bag with the target feeling in either hand, you're done.

Alternately, you can stay with just one hand and heal all of the stuck bags (ribosomes) that have the target sensation, one after another. When you can't find any more with that hand (trying to feel a bag will now be like pure imagination without any substance), then switch to the other hand and continue healing each new bag that has the same target sensation in it. But it is usually easier to switch hands back and forth after each association healing is finished – this also tends to uncover associations that were not in awareness at the start of the procedure.

Why can there be more than one bag? Since associations form during a biographical trauma moment, if there is something in the environment that is the same or similar each time, a client can have an association feeling tied to a number of damaged body genes. For example, say you were trying to heal an association to drinking beer, there might be a number of 'beer' associations from various times in your life.

In general, we need to heal only one or two target ribosomes (for example, there is only one association per ribosomal voice). But some issues can have many (up to a dozen) ribosomes that need healing. As this is uncommon, you are probably targeting bags with similar feelings rather than just the one required target feeling. If you are a therapist with a client, you need to decide if also healing them is helpful or just an irrelevant side issue.

Continue until the client cannot find any more imaginary crumpled bags that radiate the target sensation in either hand.

Step 5: Check the original issue

Since you are healing associations for a reason – such as eliminating a ribosomal voice, withdrawal or craving symptoms, or a symptom that keeps returning - check the original problem. Repeat for any new associations that are noticed. (Note to therapists: when this is complete, you might want to continue the healing on generational or biographical traumas, as described in Paula Courteau's *The Whole-Hearted Healing Workbook*.)

A final caution

Do not attempt to improve or modify this technique. It is very well tested for safety; any major modifications might trigger negative symptoms from subcellular pathogens or disturbing subcellular homeostasis.

Appendix E

The Tribal Block Technique™

This process is designed for clients who are struggling with the tribal block problem. The tribal block influences personal choices, causes people to stay within dysfunctional social roles, and act in harmful ways approved by their culture and society.

- This process is used to eliminate one tribal block issue at a time.
- Most people can use this process successfully, but it involves a (relatively short) period of relatively intense emotional suffering.
- This process should be used with a therapist, but after some initial supervision it can be used for self-help. Especially for the first few times, facing the feelings involved can be difficult without guidance.
- We haven't seen any problems with this technique, but it should be used with caution as there is a theoretical potential for stimulating cord-cutting trauma with its related suicidal feelings.
- If you currently or recently have been feeling suicidal, do *not* use this technique unless under the supervision of a therapist trained in suicide intervention.

This technique demonstrates the existence and psychological impact of a severe, very wide-spread subcellular fungal parasite infection. For a total and permanent elimination of this fungal parasite with all its tribal block problems, we currently use the regression process that is part of the Silent Mind Technique. However, it is slower, harder to do, and has more potential side effects. (For more information, see Chapters 4 and 6.)

Tribal Block Technique™
Revision 1.7, Sept 20, 2011

Step 1: Think about the issue

Have the client think about their issue. Each situation will have its own unique tribal block. We strongly recommend that the client write down their issue in a single short sentence. They want to be able to stay focused on just that one issue, and not drift to other variations or topics. If they drift, they will never finish the process, as an unending stream of emotions will continue to arise.

Surprisingly, the tribal block can be activated in nearly *any* activity in one's life. For most people, the tribal block acts to keep them in the 'status quo' or in their role in life, no matter what that situation is. Some specific issues that are almost always tribally blocked are a desire for a peak state, or taking altruistically positive actions in the world.

Because the tribal block influences many client problems and behaviors, we recommend always checking for it before starting any therapy.

Example:
A student felt intense fear as she read a book about peak states processes. The fear turned out to be the tribal block problem, as she discovered when she turned her attention out through her belly button. She used the tribal block process on reading and doing the peak states processes, and the fear vanished.

Step 2: Move the CoA behind your belly button
Move your 'center of awareness' (CoA) to just behind your belly button, as if you were looking out a keyhole or the porthole in a boat. (See Chapter 3 for a definition of the CoA). Some trauma healing may be needed to allow the client to move their CoA to the navel - techniques like EFT are often helpful. If they have trouble keeping their CoA at the belly, it is sometimes helpful to have them place their hand over their navel.

Some people have found that instead of moving their CoA to their belly button, it is more effective to leave their CoA where it is and 'move' their belly button to their CoA's location in their body. Although this sounds like it is the same procedure, people report that this works while in contrast trying to move their CoA does not.

Example:
A client had a problem with moving her CoA into her belly. It turns out that this area of her body always felt numb after she had a C-section. The client didn't realize that her CoA wasn't getting to the right location because of the numbness. Healing the C-section trauma eliminated the problem and allowed her to move her CoA to the belly button successfully.

Step 2a: Unusually severe tribal block

People who have unusually severe tribal block are often able to simply close their eyes and 'look outwardly' and sense or 'see' what feels like many people or objects. These people or objects are sending emotional feelings (that can be either positive or negative) at the client. If this is the case, skip step 2 - do not move your CoA to the belly button - and go to step 4. We currently estimate that this occurs in around 10-20% of the client population.

Caution

People who have this excessive tribal block experience should not move their CoA to the belly button area. This makes their underlying tribal block problem worse.

Step 3: Sense the emotion coming into your belly button

Once your CoA is in your belly behind the belly button, 'look' out from your belly button and sense what emotions are coming at you (into you) from the outside while you think about the issue you are trying to resolve. It's a bit like looking out a keyhole or small porthole. (Kinesthetically, it might feel like expanding from your belly button.) Many people can 'see' things out there, but this isn't necessary - the key is to sense whatever *emotions* are coming in through the belly button from the 'tribe'. Focus on feeling (or sensing, if you are kinesthetic) whatever is out there. The emotional tone can be pleasant (admiration, connection, etc), or negative (threatening, anger, rejection).

There are two sets of feelings involved with the tribal block work, and sometimes it takes some teaching to get the client to understand: the feeling that is coming from the *outside* tribe, and the response that is coming from the person's *reaction* to that external feeling coming in. Essentially, it is like working with two people – the client and a person who is trying to manipulate the client. Thus, one can 'tap' to heal one's own reaction, but one has to use Step 4 to get rid of the tribal block coming in from the outside.

In most circumstances, looking out the belly button is optimum. However, in a few cases, we've also found that some tribal blocks are being accessed in other places in the body, like the back of the neck, or chest. This rarely happens, but does occur and the student should be watching for physical sensations in the body locations due to tribal block entering in non-standard locations.

Most people also have a 'visual' component to this experience, but it is not necessary – the key is in noticing what emotions the 'tribe' is sending into you. Some of these visual clients don't see people in their field of view. Instead, they see a flat area with a large variety of things in it -

buildings, chocolate-covered melted snowmen, nature scenes, figures, objects, dark or colored areas, or borders to their vision, and so on. These are what their 'tribe' looks like to them. Whatever you see out there is radiating an emotional tone that affects you.

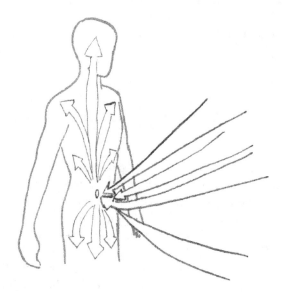

Figure E.1: The emotions coming into the navel from a borg fungus.

WARNING

Make sure the client doesn't go 'out' into the area in front of their belly - they need to stay inside themselves. Be sure to remain inside your body - do *not* go out into the area outside your belly button. This both blocks the process from working, and can also trigger long lasting problems, such as feeling one's body has become distorted or other strange and uncomfortable sensations. Stay inside yourself!

Step 3a: Trouble in sensing the tribal emotion

Some people have trouble sensing the emotions that are coming in from the 'tribe', either because the emotional tone is one that they block out due to trauma; or because they just don't know how to do this step. In this latter case, have them sense or look out the belly button 'key hole' at their immediate family and relatives. Because people commonly find their immediate family in the tribal block, this allows most people to start to sense or 'see' the source of the feelings being sent towards them. Once they have accomplished this, have them 'widen their view' out to the entire 'tribe', who will all be radiating the same emotion. (People can experience the tribal block differently. Sometimes it feels like only a single person is 'tribal blocking' them; usually there is a whole crowd; or at first there is just a single person, and when the client notices their emotional tone, a whole 'tribe' appears.)

With experience, we've found that just a few people still don't understand the instructions. The process is very simple, but some people try and make it more complicated. For example, we've seen people try to go too deeply and 'overshoot' the experience.

Some people don't have any tribal block around a given situation. In that case, the field of view is clear and white, and there is no emotional content in it.

Step 3b: Suppressing the tribal block emotions
Some clients have been so traumatized around particular feelings that they 'blank out' the emotion in the tribal block, and need help in accessing it so they can heal it. If the client is blanking out, one can still check for this because they will feel heavy (in contrast to light) as they repress and block their feelings. For example, a client could not tolerate sensing anger directed towards her; another emotional withdrawal. Fortunately, people can still see or sense that there is something out in the area of view, even though they cannot initially feel any emotional tone. Asking what emotions they can't tolerate (as might cause them to turn away from a movie scene) often works. Using EFT on their bodily reaction (to the blanked emotion coming at them) also works.

Example:
A woman who wasn't able to see, but rather was kinesthetically able to feel tribal block found herself unable to move into her belly, which wasn't normal for her. The tribal feelings coming at her were causing her to 'flee' from her belly region, and she was suppressing the feeling that was coming into her out of her conscious awareness. When she healed her resistance to that emotion, she found she could move into her belly button region again.

Step 4: Acceptance eliminates the block
The key to healing the tribal block is having the client recognize that there are two distinct emotional and physical experiences going on. The first is coming from the outside, from the 'tribe'. The second is the client's reaction to the emotion that he is receiving from the 'tribe'. These are two separate problems, although they can often be addressed together in this

process. This can be confusing for clients to understand, because they are programmed by our society to believe that anything they feel is their own feeling. It can take some patience to help them discriminate between their own feeling and the one that is coming in from the outside.

To heal the tribal block, have the client *accept and allow* all the feelings that are coming towards him from the 'tribe'. The biggest problem here is the traumatic reactions the client has to the incoming feeling. These responses can block the client's acceptance of the incoming emotion in many cases. However, often the client can temporarily 'override' their responses and still accept the incoming feeling, say by recalling a time when they were feeling very accepting or loving. If needed, use EFT or equivalent to help this process. Some clients find that using a hand pressed on their belly button helps keep their focus.

Continue to encourage the client to accept the negative feelings (or even positive ones) they feel coming towards them from the 'tribe'. Most issues have more than one emotion that needs to be faced. As one disappears, another replaces it. Sometimes this new feeling is pleasant, and the client has the temptation to quit. Don't let them! Continue to the endpoint in step 5. By analogy, the tribal block can try to control people with a stick (the painful emotions) or a carrot (the pleasant emotions).

Another person found this variation useful – she imagined that she was a hollow vessel. She let whatever radiated out from the 'tribe' pass through her and out (in her case, out her head). This is a very useful trick for this process.

Do *not* let the client get involved with communicating with or going to the 'tribe' - make sure they simply accept what the 'tribe' is feeling, and not try to manipulate it. This does not work, and just stalls the healing.

Step 4b: No end of the incoming emotions

We've occasionally seen clients who appear to have a never-ending stream of external emotions coming at them. Typically there are no more than 4 or 5 different feelings in a row that come at them around their issue, but for some issues in some people there can be more than 5. However, this problem is usually caused by their loss of focus on the original issue, and they've started to think about new issues, with entirely new tribal block feelings.

Step 5: The process endpoint

As the client continues to accept the incoming emotions, they will notice a heaviness and pressure on their body decreasing as they start to eliminate the last emotional tone. Virtually everyone doesn't realize that the heavy, pressing down sensation was there all the time, until it starts to fade.

Continue accepting until the pressure completely vanishes. For some who have been battling a long standing tribal block issue, this can feel like suddenly taking off a heavy backpack: "When I first did this, I spent the rest of the day feeling like I had just been let out for summer vacation."

As they continue to think about the issue, all incoming emotions should also vanish. As a check, they should expand their awareness to include their family's homeland, and continue to expand their awareness to all of humanity. All feelings of pressure should be gone, and all external emotions should also be gone.

In people who can 'see' out their belly button, they should continue healing until all the objects, colors, or figures vanish. Even metaphoric images like trees, landscape, faint patches of mist or vapor need to be accepted and dissolved. The endpoint to the process occurs when only a clear white field is left is their entire field of view. Finally, do not let them move out into the white field to look more closely – this can trigger other problems.

A final caution

Do not attempt to improve or modify this technique. It is very well tested for safety; any major modifications might trigger negative symptoms from subcellular pathogens or disturb subcellular homeostasis.

Glossary

Associational trauma: Two or more feelings or sensations that are coupled together during a moment of trauma. (As in Pavlov's dog associating the sound of a bell with the taste of food.)

Biographical trauma: A traumatic experience during one's lifetime; this includes egg and sperm trauma.

Body brain: The reptilian brain, at the base of the skull. It thinks in gestalt body sensations (called the 'felt sense' in Gendlin's Focusing), and experiences itself in the lower belly. It is called the *hara* in Japanese. It is the brain that we communicate with when doing dowsing or muscle testing. At the subcellular level, it is the endoplasmic reticulum.

Body associations: The body brain makes non-logical associations during traumas that then direct its actions later in life. For example, this is the basis of the 'Pavlov's dog' connecting a bell sound with food.

Brains: Refers to different portions of the brain that have separate self-awareness: the mind (primate) heart (mammalian), and body (reptilian) of the triune brain model. Their awarenesses are extensions of the organelles' inside the primary cell, which in turn are extensions of the sacred being blocks. Also refers to the extended triune brain model: perineum, body, solar plexus, heart, mind, third eye, crown, navel (placenta) and spine (sperm tail).

CoA (Center of Awareness): Using a finger, you can find your center of awareness by pointing at where 'you' are in your body. Can be at a particular point, or diffuse, or in more than one location, or both internal to the body and external.

Cords: It describes a dysfunctional connection between two people (actually, between a trauma in each person) that can be seen as a 'tube' or 'cord'. These cause the real-time sensation that others have a 'personality' (emotional tone) when one thinks about them. It is actually tentacles of a fungal organism that penetrates the cell.

Coalescence: The precellular organelles combine to form a primordial germ cell at the coalescence stage. This occurs inside the parent who is still a blastocyst inside the grandmother.

Copies: A duplicate of someone else's emotions or sensations on one's own body. Copies are caused by a bacterial species that lives in the cytoplasm.

Differential diagnosis: When a symptom can have different causes, the therapist narrows down to the real cause by checking to see if other symptoms match one of the possible choices.

DPR (Distant Personality Release): A Peak States technique that eliminates transference and counter-transference between people by dissolving 'cords' (and the corresponding traumas) between them.

EFT (Emotional Freedom Technique): A therapy that uses tapping on meridian points to eliminate emotional and physical discomfort. Classified as a power therapy, in the subcategory of 'energy' or 'meridian' therapy.

EMDR (Eye Movement Desensitization and Reprocessing): A regression trauma healing therapy involving the repeated movement of attention from left to right, either with the eyes or by touching the body on alternate sides.

Epigenetic damage: The inherited problem of a gene not working properly ('inhibited gene expression') even though there is nothing wrong with the gene's DNA. Psychologically, this is experienced as generational trauma.

ER (endoplasmic reticulum): A folded membrane subcellular structure attached to the nucleus in the cell cytoplasm. Rough ER has pores with ribosomes embedded in them; smooth ER does not. This organelle is a part of the body brain consciousness.

Gaia commands: Developmental events can be broken down into biological steps, with each step being described by a short phrase. In regression, these phrases are experienced as commands sent from an external source we call Gaia, the living self-aware biosphere of our planet, which guides our development in real-time.

Gene expression: When a protein is needed in the cell, a gene is moved out of storage in the nucleolus and a messenger RNA copy made. This mRNA string is then sent into the cytoplasm to be 'read' by a ribosome and a protein made.

Generational trauma: Subcellular structural problems passed down through the family line. They cause emotions that feel very 'personal', that something is very wrong with oneself. They can be eliminated with a variety of techniques.

Heart brain: The limbic system, or old mammalian brain. It thinks in sequences of emotions, and experiences itself in the center of the chest.

Histone: Any of a group of proteins found in chromatin. In this text, we focus on the histone that covers DNA gene, looking like plastic insulation on a wire.

mRNA (messenger ribonucleic acid): It is an RNA copy of a nuclear DNA gene that is sent out into the cytoplasm. This mRNA string contains the information needed for a ribosome to make a specific protein.

Muscle testing: Communicating with the body consciousness by using muscle strength as an indicator. Same mechanism as applied kinesiology, and the terms are used interchangeably.

NLP (Neurolinguistic Programming): A collection of techniques for healing or communication. This un-trademarked term does not have any clear meaning because there is no agreement on what the techniques are or their content.

Nuclear core: A hollow volume inside the nucleolus, containing fundamental structures of consciousness.

Nuclear pores: Openings in the nuclear membrane that have sphincters in them that resemble camera irises. There are 4-5,000 pores in the primary cell nucleus.

OBE (Out of Body Experience): A person's awareness can move outside their body. This phenomenon is most easily noticed in trauma memories that are 'seen' from an OBE perspective.

Organelle: The different types of structures inside a cell that act like various 'organs'.

Organelle brains: The self-aware organelles in the sperm, egg, or fertilized cell. There are seven self-aware organelles in the sperm or egg, and nine compounded organelles in zygote and adult cells. They share consciousness with their corresponding multi-celled triune brains. This label is usually shortened to just 'organelle' in the context of self-aware cell structures.

Peak experience: A short-lived, unusually good feeling that enhances functionality in the world.

Peak state: A stable, long lasting peak experience of one of over a hundred different types. These range from exceptional physical abilities to continuously positive feelings to experiences outside the Western belief system.

Personality: This is what others sense about a person when they turn their attention to them. Rather than being a mental construct in the observer, it is a real-time experience of particular traumas in the one being observed. It is caused by the borg fungus. The DPR process is used to dissolve this connection.

Power therapy: A phrase coined by Dr. Figley who also originated the psychological category called post traumatic stress disorder (PTSD). It applies to extremely effective therapies (originally EMDR, TIR, TFT, and VKD) that remove symptoms from PTSD and other issues.

Precellular organelles: The self-aware organelles before they combine to form a primordial germ cell. The different types are identified either by their biological name in the cell, or by the triune brain they share a continuity of awareness with (e.g., body, heart, etc.).

Precellular trauma: Trauma that occurs to precellular organelles.

Primary cell: The only cell in the body that contains consciousness. It acts as the master pattern for all other cells. Formed at the forth cell division after conception.

Primordial germ cell (PGC): The original cell that eventually matures into a sperm or egg. They are first formed in the parental blastocyst shortly after implantation inside the grandmother.

Psychosis: The client has lost contact with external reality. Many very different and unrelated problems are labeled this way.

PTSD (Post Traumatic Stress Disorder): This is the standard name for severe, long-lasting reactions to traumatic events.

Ribosome: Found in large numbers floating in the cell cytoplasm, they look a bit like crumpled-up bags. Made of ribosomal RNA and proteins, they manufacture proteins based on information from mRNA strings.

Soul loss: A phrase used in shamanism describing pieces of self-awareness that have left the person. This person will typically feel lonely, sad, and miss the person who triggered this problem.

Spiritual emergency: An experience from various spiritual, mystical or shamanic traditions that becomes a crisis. This is not the same as a crisis of faith.

Subcellular psychobiology: Many psychological (and physical) symptoms are directly caused by various biological disorders, parasites or pathogens inside the cell. Subcellular problems can be treated with various psychological-like techniques that directly interact with subcellular structures; or with trauma-healing techniques that repair early developmental damage that directly or indirectly caused subsequent subcellular issues.

SUDS (Subjective Units of Distress Scale): A relative measure used to evaluate the degree of pain or emotional discomfort. Originally from a scale of 1 to 10, common usage is now from 0 (no pain) to 10 (as much pain as it's possible to have).

TIR (Traumatic Incident Reduction): An excellent power therapy that uses regression.

Trauma: A moment in time, or string of moments when sensations, emotions, and thoughts are stored from painful, difficult or pleasurable experiences. They cause problems because they make fixed beliefs that guide behavior inappropriately. Severe trauma creates post-traumatic stress disorder.

Tribal block: The influence of culture in people. It also causes cultural conflicts and hostility between members of different cultures. Caused by a fungus.

Triune brain: The full name is the "Papez-MacLean triune brain model". The brain is built out of three major, separate biological structures formed in evolution. They are the R-complex (body), the limbic system (heart), and the neocortex (mind). Each is self-aware, built for different functions, and thinks by using either sensations, feelings, or thoughts. They generate the phenomenon of the subconscious. With a certain peak state they can be communicated with directly.

WHH (Whole-Hearted Healing): A regression therapy technique. It uses awareness of the out-of-body experience ("dissociation") associated with trauma to heal.

Index

D

E

F

G

Q

qualifications · 133
qualifications of therapist · 133

R

racing thoughts · 77
racism's fungal cause · 53
recreational drugs · 93
referrals · 137
regression · 70
    changing the past · 72
    Whole-Hearted Healing · 10
reporter voice · 105
reptilian brain · 34
research
    breakthrough mindsets · 7
    multi-disciplinary · 7
    non-publication · 91
    prototype development · 119
    risk management · 98
    risks · 96
    safety protocols · 97
    working in · xi
resilience · 6
ribosomal voices · 34, 37
    and schizophrenia treatments · 79
    average number · 81
    diagnosis · 76
    fixed locations in space · 107
    speaking foreign languages · 61
    steps for elimination of · 139
ribosomes · 55
    containing trauma feelings · 36
    containing voices · 37
    in the ER · 75
risks · 87
    Body Association Technique · 88
    management · 98
    of self-experimentation · xxi
    of therapy · 135
    research · 96
    Silent Mind Technique · 89
    with peak states processes · 136
Rogerian therapy · 14

S

safety alerts · 99
safety issues · xxi
safety, feeling of · 121
Salier, Samsara · xvi, 99
schizophrenia
    and Silent Mind Technique · 131
    ribosomal voice treatment impact · 79
Schizophrenia Society of Canada · 43
schizophrenia symptoms · 42
schizotypal disorders (F21) · 80
self-help · 95
self-mutilation clients · 94
self-talk · 107
sex addiction · 78
    and voices · 23
sexual attractions · 76, 89
    and voices · 21
    steps for elimination of · 140
shard · 59
side-effects · 130
Silent Mind Technique · 38, 70
    effectiveness · 83
    how long? · 129
    pay for results contract · 127
    vs Body Association Technique · 76
smoke cloud hallucination
    as a ribosomal voice · 38
solar plexus and peak states · 45
Sorensen, Kate · 29
soul loss · 17, 89
soul stealing · 17
sound loops · 108
spirit communication · 15
spiritual emergencies · 9, 93
spiritual experiences · 14
spiritual realm
    as subcellular view · 31
spouse's reactions · 90
stigma of hearing voices · xix
stress and voices · 81
subcellular psychobiology
    effects of various diseases · 81
    new field · xix
subvocalization · 107, 129
SUDS (Subjective Units of Distress Scale) · 107
suicidal client · 90, 94